FIRST AID HINTS FOR THE HORSE OWNER
A Veterinary Note Book

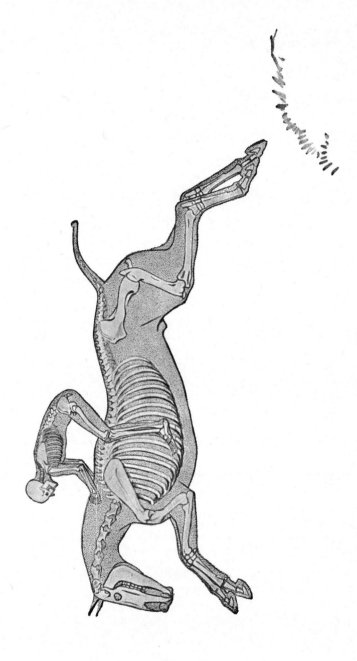

DIAGRAM OF A MAN AND HORSE ILLUSTRATING THE POSITION OF THE BONES WHILST JUMPING.

FIRST AID HINTS FOR

THE HORSE OWNER

A Veterinary Note Book

LT.-COL. W. E. LYON

Illustrated by
HUMPHREY DIXON

COLLINS
ST. JAMES'S PLACE LONDON

First published by Constable, 1933
Second edition, Revised 1950
Third impression   *1951*
Fourth impression   *1955*
Fifth impression   *1957*
Sixth impression   *1959*
Seventh impression   *1962*
Eighth impression   *1963*
Ninth impression   *1965*
Tenth impression   *1966*
Eleventh impression   *1968*
Twelfth impression   *1969*
Thirteenth impression   *1971*
Reprinted   *1972*
Reprinted   *1978*

ISBN 0 00 211251 5
Made and Printed in Great Britain by
William Collins Sons & Co Ltd Glasgow

Contents

CHAP.   PAGE

    Author's Foreword to first edition   9
    Introduction to new edition   11
  I STABLE MANAGEMENT   13
    Care of Hunters   13
    Hunting Off Grass   25
    Care of Saddlery   29
 II LAMENESS   37
III INJURIES   69
 IV SKIN DISEASES   81
  V INTERNAL DISEASES   90
 VI WIND, HEART AND EYE   112
VII TEETH   119
VIII BREEDING   125
    Appendix   133
    Index   149

AUTHOR'S FOREWORD
TO THE FIRST EDITION

WHEN I undertook to produce this book I did so with a light heart, having the greatest confidence in the technical knowledge and literary ability of my friend and collaborator Colonel Hugh Jagger.

One day we made out our list of contents; a few days later—quite suddenly—he died. This, I am convinced, was the only unkind thing he ever did in his life.

His ready sympathy, his sense of humour and his understanding of our troubles must have left a lifelong impression on the memory of those who were fortunate enough to come in contact with him, whether professionally or in private life.

It was not until, left to myself, I started to write this book that I realised how numerous were the diseases that could render our mutual friend the horse temporarily or permanently useless to man.

More poignantly still I realised, in spite of my long association with horses, how meagre was my knowledge of their various ailments.

It was the very early realisation of this deficiency that confirmed my resolution to seek the aid of some of the most expert veterinary surgeons in the country. To those, therefore, who have most kindly helped me by their criticisms of my efforts I am more grateful than I can express. This book is the richer for many practical and useful hints, thanks to Mr. L. F. Hill, Mr. Ernest Clipston and Mr. H. Oldham.

My last acknowledgments I am keeping for Captain Jack Grant-Ives and Captain Humphrey Dixon, without whose timely help at the most critical stage and up to the time of its going to the printers this book would not now be in your hands.

For those who wish to probe deeper into the knowledge of veterinary science I recommend Black's *Veterinary Dictionary*, Fitzwygram's *Horses and Stables*, and Hayes' *Veterinary Notes for Horse Owners*, which have been invaluable to me as books of reference.

Just as no medical treatise could possibly take the place of your local practitioner or surgeon, so this book makes no claim to deputise for your veterinary surgeon. I dare to hope, however, that it may prove to be an efficient understudy where professional aid is neither an urgent necessity nor perhaps easily procurable.

1933.   W. E. L.

INTRODUCTION
TO NEW EDITION

It is sixteen years since this book was first published. It went out of print and before it could be reprinted a German airman dropped a bomb on it, and that was that!

One of the very few good effects of the War has been to drive more and more people into the company of horses, the majority of whom have, of necessity, to look after them unaided by such luxuries as grooms: it is this fact that has spurred me on to revising this book.

A World War, in spite of all its miseries and horrors, undoubtedly acts as a forcing house for scientific research and in spite of the fact that early in the War the exhilarating sound of horses' hooves was ruthlessly replaced by the clanging and roaring of mechanised vehicles, nevertheless veterinary science kept marching on.

What was more natural, therefore, when I was looking for somebody to hold my hand and guide my pen along the right lines, than to turn to an old friend, Colonel C. H. S. Townsend, who was himself a pioneer in veterinary research in the Middle East and who helped me with the original version of the book. Without his wholehearted assistance and up-to-date veterinary knowledge I would never have had a hope of bringing out this new edition.

Finally, I am glad to say that Captain Humphrey Dixon, who originally illustrated the book, was at hand to add a few more drawings. This was lucky for few artists possess such fundamental knowledge of the anatomy of the horse or can impart it with such economy of line. To these two friends I am, once more, eternally grateful.

1949.   W.E.L.

CHAPTER I

STABLE MANAGEMENT

CARE OF HUNTERS

HORSES confined in stables are being kept under artificial conditions, and in consequence skill is required to maintain them in good health. Living under natural conditions the horse eats grass; he eats for a very considerable number of hours each day and during the night; he feeds in small quantities at frequent intervals, and he drinks whenever he feels inclined. He has a very small stomach for his size. These facts should be borne in mind when horses are in the stable, and the less the natural conditions are disturbed the better.

Conditioning. Horses intended for hunting during the season should be brought in from grass during July or, at the latest, August. During July the grass begins to lack the nutritive qualities which it had in May and June, and the horse will come up in less soft condition if he has been given a feed of 5 lb. oats daily the last few weeks at grass. This extra condition is due partly to the hard food and partly to the fact that the oats give the horse more energy and that he therefore takes more exercise on his own.

Great care must be taken when the horse is brought in that he does not take cold and start coughing. During the first week in the stable he should not be made to sweat, and the top door of the stable should be kept open night and day to give all possible air. Nothing is more likely to start a cough than a stuffy stable.

During the first week in the stable the horse should be given damp bran and hay with little or no oats. The

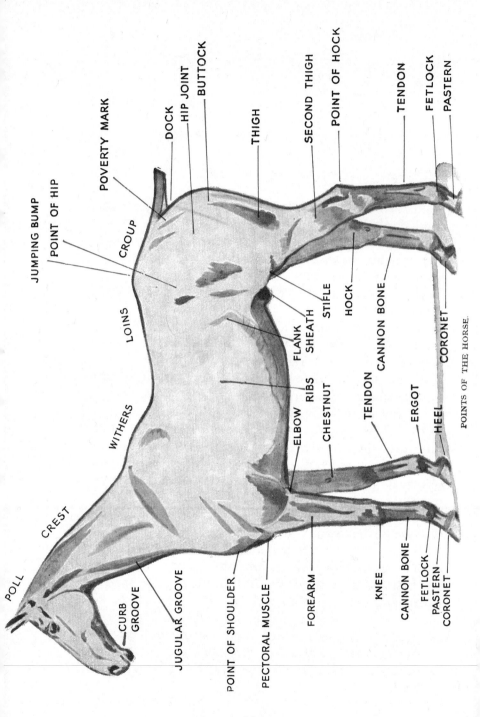

POINTS OF THE HORSE.

POLL

CREST

WITHERS

LOINS

CROUP

JUMPING BUMP

POINT OF HIP

POVERTY MARK

DOCK

HIP JOINT

BUTTOCK

THIGH

SECOND THIGH

POINT OF HOCK

TENDON

FETLOCK

PASTERN

STIFLE

HOCK

CANNON BONE

FLANK

SHEATH

RIBS

ELBOW

CHESTNUT

TENDON

ERGOT

HEEL

CORONET

CURB GROOVE

JUGULAR GROOVE

POINT OF SHOULDER

PECTORAL MUSCLE

FOREARM

KNEE

CANNON BONE

FETLOCK

PASTERN

CORONET

14

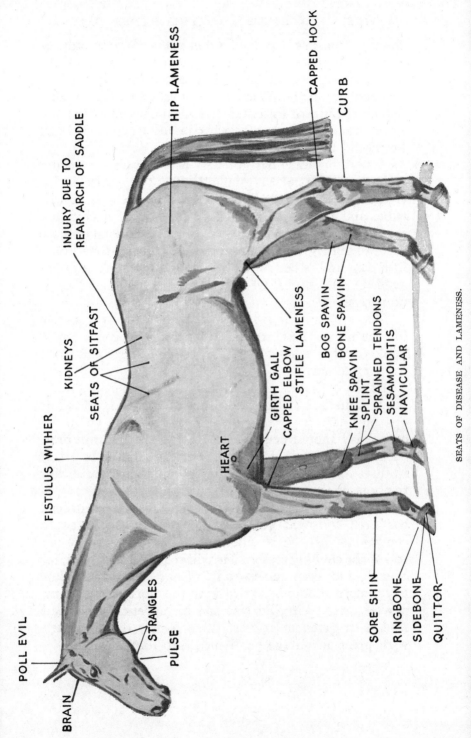

POLL EVIL
BRAIN
STRANGLES
PULSE
FISTULUS WITHER
INJURY DUE TO REAR ARCH OF SADDLE
KIDNEYS
SEATS OF SITFAST
HIP LAMENESS
CAPPED HOCK
CURB
HEART
GIRTH GALL
CAPPED ELBOW
STIFLE LAMENESS
BOG SPAVIN
BONE SPAVIN
KNEE SPAVIN
SPLINT
SPRAINED TENDONS
SESAMOIDITIS
NAVICULAR
SORE SHIN
RINGBONE
SIDEBONE
QUITTOR

SEATS OF DISEASE AND LAMENESS.

15

change from grass to dry food is likely to cause indigestion and diarrhœa. If at the end of the first week the diarrhœa persists, the horse should be given bran mashes for twenty-four hours and then physicked with an aloes ball or 1½ pints of linseed oil. If the horse comes up from grass in poor condition, worms should be suspected and he should be treated accordingly.

When the horse has got well over the physic the oat ration may be raised gradually as the exercise is increased. Plenty of walking exercise is essential at this time, and the owner need have no fear of giving too much of it. The horse when out at grass takes slow exercise during the larger part of the twenty-four hours in a day, and is better for plenty of slow exercise when stabled. He probably enjoys it, as confinement is unnatural.

The longer that slow work is continued the better for the horse. Fast exercise when in gross condition is liable to affect a horse's wind, damage his legs and work irreparable harm.

As the horse becomes fit, slow trotting exercise should be given and steady trots uphill are excellent for muscling up the quarters. With this exercise about 8-10 lb. of oats a day should be sufficient with 2 lb. of damp bran added and about 14 lb. of hay. The corn should be given in three feeds, a little of the hay given after exercise and the bulk of the hay last thing at night.

Feeding when in Hard Work. If this treatment has been followed your horse should be in first-rate condition when he is called upon for fast work at the end of the cubbing season. He will require about 10-14 lb. of oats, 2 lb. bran and 12-16 lb. of hay daily. The quantity of corn should be varied with the work that is being expected from him, his size and his appetite. The food should be given in at least three feeds a day and may with great advantage be divided into four meals.

Many stud grooms like to give their horses a feed late in the evening before a day's hunting, and the author likes this feed given every evening.

A horse will consume a larger quantity of oats in a day if they are given in many small feeds than if given in a few larger ones, and this fact is to be borne in mind when there is a delicate feeder in the stable.

A delicate feeder must never be offered any more than he will take, and if he does not clear up, the surplus should be removed at once.

The quality of the oats should also receive the attention of the horse owner. Oats are sold by the hundredweight or by the quarter, which consists of two sacks of 12 stone each. They should be hard and dry and should smell sweet. White oats are generally preferred by hunting men, but grey and black are both good provided they are heavy. Twelve stone of oats in a sack may fill the sack so that it is quite difficult to tie up the neck, or the sack may only appear about three-quarters full; if the sack appears brim full, the oats will be quite useless for feeding hunters as they contain far too great a proportion of husk, which is valueless.

New oats are not digestible and should not be fed before Christmas. It is not easy to distinguish between old and new oats, so the safest method is to buy sufficient oats to last you till Christmas just before harvest time.

Some horses do not digest whole oats well, and for these it is advisable to have them lightly rolled. Rolled oats are far more bulky weight for weight than whole oats; one sack of whole oats equalling about one and a half of rolled.

First-rate hay is quite as important as good oats. It should have a pleasant smell, be dry, and green to light brown in colour. Hay which is produced from temporary pastures and contains a mixture of clover and rye grass or sainfoin and rye grass is better for horses than the softer hay which is grown on permanent pastures.

To be good, hay must have been cut early in the season, preferably before the middle of June, and got into stack without rain or too much handling. After this time the seeds begin to drop out of the hay and the consistency of the stalks becomes more like straw.

A small proportion of the hay should be chaffed and given mixed with each feed, and the long hay may be given on the ground or in a hay net. The use of a hay net is economical as it prevents the hay being trampled in with the bedding and wasted.

Bran is another safe and useful food for horses. About 2 lb. a day mixed with the oat feed assists digestion. It is somewhat constipating if given dry and a mild laxative when given damp. It may therefore be used to regulate the bowels.

Bran mash is always given to horses on their return home from a hard day's work as it is easily digested. Linseed gruel should be added to it.

A bran mash is made as follows: Fill half a bucket full of bran and add enough boiling water to damp the whole. Stir it well with a stick until all is damp and cover the bucket with a sack. After it has steamed for about half an hour it will be cool enough for a horse to eat. A few rolled oats and a pound of linseed which has been simmering all day on the hob will greatly increase the palatability of the mash.

Bran mash is also given on Saturday night, and as the horse will probably not be at work on Sunday, $\frac{1}{4}$ lb. of Epsom salts should be added to it on this occasion.

Rock salt should be available for horses to lick, and most horses like it.

Beans are a very heating food for a horse and must never be given unless a horse is in hard work. Towards the end of a hunting season a handful of cracked beans the day before hunting will undoubtedly help to keep a horse in good fettle.

Barley which has been boiled may be given to a horse in limited quantities. It is useful for getting a bit of flesh on a poor animal.

A child's pony should have very little or no oats given to it as it is essential that it should be quiet and not play up. It is really far better left at grass with hay and bran as an extra.

Watering. The watering of horses is a subject on which a variety of opinions exists, but the author likes to follow nature as closely as possible and leaves water in the box day and night. A horse should not do fast work immediately after a drink or a heavy feed, so many grooms do not give a hunter much water before a day's hunting, but if he has had water with him throughout the night, he will not drink too much in the morning if it is left in the box.

The water should be changed morning and evening.

Another question which is controversial is whether to allow a horse to drink when he comes in hot. The author's opinion is "Let him drink," and he has never known a horse to suffer from it.

By far the best method is to have automatic water bowls fitted into each loose-box. Horses learn how to use them within twenty-four hours; they are a great saving of labour added to which the horse gets his water whenever he feels inclined without gulping it down too rapidly.

Grooming. Grooming is a further subject of importance, and the adage that good grooming is as important as good feeding is true.

The dandy brush is used for removing rough mud, and must be used gently on horses with tender skins when they have been clipped.

The body brush does the main work. The groom

should stand well back from the horse and lean the weight of his body on to the brush, which should penetrate to the skin. It is worked in the direction that the coat lies. By its action the grease is removed from the skin and the pores rendered more open to exude sweat when work is being done. The brush is kept clean with the curry comb, and this should be the only function of the curry comb in grooming.

The water brush has longer hairs than the body brush. It is used for the mane and tail, and is also admirably adapted for the dry brushing of the head and legs.

A hoof pick is another essential tool which cannot be used too frequently when a horse is in the stable.

A sweat-scraper is useful when a horse is brought in hot or when he comes in very wet.

Straw wisps and hard hay wisps are also used for drying and stimulating the skin and acting as a massage to the muscles.

The stable rubber, which is a great favourite among grooms, is nothing but a duster. It may be used to give a final polish to the coat, but it does not take the place of a body brush, and its excessive use is to be deprecated.

The principal grooming of the day should take place after work, and a thorough grooming will take one man an hour. A brisk grooming gives the skin a healthy glow in the same way as the brisk rub of a Turkish towel does to a man.

Grooming of this kind diminishes the chance of a horse breaking out into a cold sweat.

The eyes, nostrils and dock should be cleaned with a moist sponge each time the horse is groomed.

Every week the sheath should be cleaned with a sponge and water.

When a horse returns from work the girths should

be loosened, the saddle raised and replaced, and the girths again done up slackly. The groom should water the horse, do the other parts and then remove the saddle. By this time the back will have cooled down slowly, regained circulation and be ready for grooming.

Quartering is an abbreviated form of grooming in which the roller is not removed. The eyes, nose and dock are sponged and the rugs turned back so that the quarters and then the forehand can be groomed.

The feet should be picked out at least twice a day, and particularly if the horse is bedded on peat or sawdust.

A common vice of grooms is the washing of a horse's legs. This should never be allowed as it is most likely to cause mud fever and cracked heels. When a horse comes in with wet, muddy legs the rough mud should be removed with a straw wisp and the legs loosely bandaged with flannel bandages. Next day the mud should be brushed out with a dry brush.

As a preventive of mud fever it is advisable to smear the back of the fetlock and heels with vaseline before hunting in wet weather.

The shoes should be inspected daily to see that they are tight and should be removed every four weeks at least and replaced or renewed.

Clipping. During the autumn when faster work is required of a horse he will be found to sweat profusely, and must be clipped or he will lose flesh rapidly. It is desirable to postpone clipping till as late in September as is practicable. The horse is apt to come out patchy if the coat is not well set before he is clipped. To look smart a horse has to be clipped at least every three weeks until Christmas, but they vary very much in the amount of coat they grow. Controversy exists as to the advisability of clipping the legs. In all horses except thoroughbreds the legs should be clipped on the first two occasions when clipping takes place. (See diagram, page 26.)

If the hair be left too thick on the legs it is impossible for the groom to discover thorns and minor scratches, and if they be clipped out through the season the likelihood of mud fever and cracked heels is increased. A mean must therefore be struck. Special clipping knives with coarse blades can be purchased for the legs which clip about twice as long as the ordinary blade, and these are sometimes useful.

Saddle marks should not be left the first time of clipping unless the horse is to be ridden side-saddle. When they are left they should be in the natural position of the saddle. Nothing looks worse than a saddle mark in the position where a saddle should go and the saddle a foot in front of it.

Feeding when not in Work. During a spell of frosty weather, or in other conditions when exercise is curtailed, the oat ration of horses which are in hard condition must be reduced, and if a frost appears likely to be prolonged a mild laxative such as a Cupis ball may be given with advantage. Over-feeding and under-exercise is the cause of Azoturia (Monday morning disease), which is sometimes fatal.

Care of the Horse when Exhausted. After hard work, such as a day's hunting, when the horse is very tired, he should be finished off as soon as possible and left quiet.

After a bucket of warm gruel which is made of well-boiled linseed thinned down in warm water, two grooms should be put to do him if possible. His legs should be bandaged with loose flannel bandages and he should be groomed down and rugged up. A linseed mash* should be given, and later in the evening a dry feed and hay.

The feeds should not be large, as a big feed may put off a very tired horse.

* See Appendix, page 142.

The horse may show symptoms of distress. He will stand with his head down, his legs straddled, and tremble. The pulse will be weak.

In this case he should be given the following "pick-me-up" :—

Aromatic spirit of Ammonia	- 2 tablespoons.
Cold water - - - - -	1 pint.

This is a good drench to keep in the stable and if the horse is no better it can be repeated in two hours' time.

Let the horse drink as much warm linseed gruel as he will.

Dry him all over carefully, especially the ears and legs. Rug him up well and bandage all four legs. Put down an ample amount of straw to encourage him to lie down.

He may then be given a warm bran mash and feed if he will eat them.

Roughing-off. As soon as the hunting season is finished those horses which are not wanted for further work should be roughed off.

The top half of the box door should be left open if this has not been done throughout the winter and plenty of air given. Draughts must, however, be avoided. The rugs should be reduced in number gradually, having regard to the temperature outside and the condition of the horse, until in about a fortnight he should do without any rugs at all. The oat ration should be cut down to 3 or 4 lb. a day and the majority of the food consist of hay and damp bran.

Grooming should cease, to allow the grease to rise in the coat, but the feet must be regularly picked out and the eyes, nose and dock sponged daily.

Turning out to Grass. After about three weeks of

this treatment the horse is ready to be turned out as soon as there is enough grass, which in many seasons is not till the second week in May in the Midlands.

Before going out the horse's legs should receive any veterinary treatment they may need, such as blistering, and the day before turning out the shoes should be removed and the feet rasped round by a blacksmith. If the fore feet are brittle, tips may be advisable, and in any case the feet should be regularly examined for split hoof while the animal is out. Splits soon spread, and "a stitch in time saves nine."

If it is an exceptionally dry summer and the ground gets hard, horses at grass often go very " feeling," especially in front.

In this case it pays to have shoes put on in front which will prevent broken hoofs and save many a lost shoe later on in the hunting season.

It is not advisable to have shoes put on behind when at grass owing to the danger of kicks.

Opinions vary as to the treatment immediately preceding going out. Many owners like their horses to go out with an empty stomach as they are less likely to gallop madly about. This is perfectly sound, but if the pasture on which the horse is to be turned out is rich and full of grass, it is then better to turn him out with a full belly so that the horse does not over-gorge himself with grass.

Lard rubbed well over the back and loins before the horse is turned out acts as a protection against the weather.

A hovel in the field is frequently used by a horse as a protection against flies but seldom against storms. The doorway and roof of the hovel must be high enough to avoid risk of injury, or it is better to be without it.

Running or spring water is desirable. Ponds are a hotbed of disease and should be avoided.

In very hot weather when flies are troublesome it is advisable to bring the horses in in the daytime and turn them out at night. They must jar their legs very considerably on hard ground kicking at flies.

At the end of June it is worth while to give a feed of oats daily as the grass goes off until the time when the horses are again brought up.

Summering Indoors. If it is desired to summer a horse in a yard or box the preparation is the same, but the horse is kept in rough instead of being let out. Four or five lbs. of oats a day may be given, but the majority of the food should consist of mown grass, vetches, lucerne and hay. The feet should be picked out as thrush may follow this method of summering unless attention is given to this point.

The horse summered in a yard will not come up in as soft condition as if he had been summered out.

July brings us to the end of the circle and the horses are brought up again.

HUNTING OFF GRASS

That horses can be hunted off grass and with their long coats on has been proved during and since the Second World War. For the majority of those wishing to follow hounds it was Hobson's Choice owing to lack of forage, grooms, and/or time to spend on feeding and exercising. That it is not a wholly satisfactory or enjoyable way of going hunting has also been proved by the number of people who, when these obstacles were able to be overcome, reverted to the older order of things.

Let us consider the advantages and disadvantages under different headings.

Food. It by no means rules out the necessity of feeding, as a horse cannot be expected to go to the end

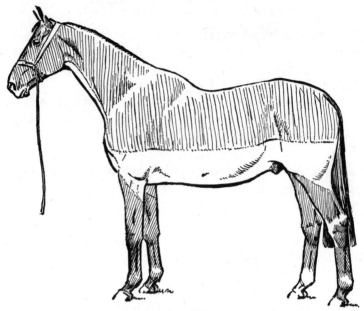

TRACE-CLIPPED.

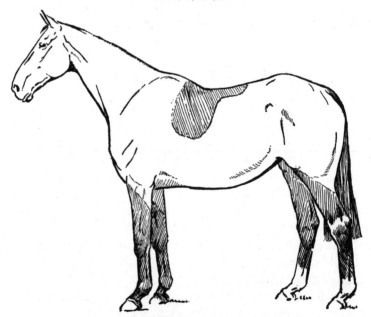

LEGS AND SADDLE MARK.

26

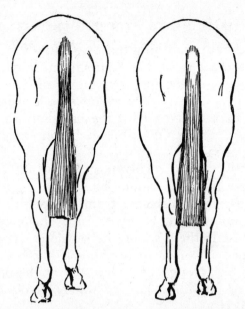

TWO WAYS OF PULLING AND CUTTING HUNTERS' TAILS.
A general rule as to length is that when the tail is " carried "
the bottom of it is level with the point of the hock.

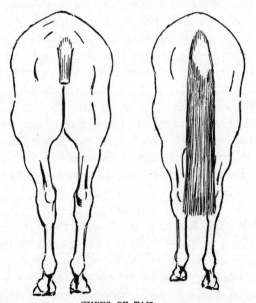

TYPES OF TAIL.
The short tail or " Cocktail."   The Racehorse's tail.

of a good hunt on nothing but a bellyful of grass, added to which there is very little nourishment in winter grass so the same amount (or even more) of oats and hay should be given. Crushed beans (about 2 lb.) and crushed or flaked maize mixed with the oats help to keep the horse warm. So, as far as forage is concerned, there is no saving of money.

Choice of Field. The most important consideration is that the field should be as dry under foot as possible, have good shelter from the prevailing wind and the feeds should be given in a sheltered spot—a covered shed if there should be such luxury as this is a help when it comes to catching a horse.

Water. A trough on a dry part of the field is the best way of providing it with water. Avoid a muddy pond at all costs.

Before and After Hunting. Many people like to bring their hunter in the night before hunting so that the accumulation of several days mud can be more easily knocked off it, in which case it is obviously necessary to have some form of stabling however rough, but, if it is brought in, it must be where it will have plenty of air otherwise it is almost certain to start coughing. However little time there is for grooming before hunting it is essential that the part to be covered by the saddle and girths should be well dried and free from mud. After hunting, providing the horse is brought in quite cool, it can be turned out at once but not fed for another half-hour otherwise colic may result.

Exercise. A horse will be all the fitter for a little exercise between hunting days, especially if he is only hunted once a week—but it is not absolutely necessary.

Clipping and New Zealand Rugs. Except in the case of a thoroughbred or when a New Zealand rug is used, it helps to keep condition on a horse if it is clipped trace high, say twice before December 1st and not again.

(See illustration on Page 26.) In any case the legs are better left unclipped and the heels untrimmed to avoid cracked heels. The mane, if any, is better left long for the sake of extra warmth: the tail is better not pulled but cut to just above the point of the hock, otherwise it is almost certain to get caked with mud. Opinions as to the usefulness of the New Zealand rug vary so much that it is difficult to know whether to recommend its use or not. Certainly it is a comfort to a horse with a fine coat and it is so made that it cannot slip round: on the other hand, unless special care is taken it may cause sore withers, or rub the back where the roller lies over the spine. A night's rain on a dry rug can make a lot of difference to its fit by the morning, so a good deal of supervision is necessary.

Health. Generally speaking, a horse is healthier out at grass than in the stable. Coughs and colds are rare: cuts and injuries heal quicker. Mud fever and cracked heels, curiously enough, are more common in the stable than out at grass. As a horse grows a thick protective coat when running out in the winter a keen lookout must be kept for lice, expecially in the second half of the season. Rain rash is also fairly common in thin-skinned horses in a very wet season. In this complaint the hair on the loins and quarters becomes matted and falls out. Dressing with cod liver oil is a good preventative and also a cure.

CARE OF SADDLERY

First of all it must be stressed that it is a very false form of economy to buy anything but saddles and bridles made of the best English leather, and having bought them it pays to look after them.

Cleaning a bridle is rather an exasperating job for it entails dismantling the whole outfit before you start and

cleaning each piece separately. Having done this, all the
bits and pieces have to be put together again.

The method of cleaning is simplicity itself. Here is
the order of procedure.

(1) Dismantle the bridle.

(2) Wash all mud and sweat marks off with warm
soft water.

(3) Leave it to dry (not near a fire) or rub it over with
a "shammy" leather till about dry.

(4) Rub in saddle soap (the best you can get).

(5) Clean the steel work. Stainless steal will save
endless labour.

Neatsfoot oil is used for keeping the leather soft so is
especially useful if the bridles are not to be used for
some time. It is also a good thing to use it on the inside
of the flaps of the saddle occasionally to keep them
supple.

A word about the linings of the saddle. Naturally
after coming in from exercise or hunting the lining will
be damp and possibly dirty due to the sweat from the
horse's back. If the saddle is left to dry in the sun or
saddle room in that condition the lining will get hard
and perhaps be the cause of a sore back; it is therefore
best to scrub the lining with warm water and leave it
to dry slowly in a warm room or in the sun.

The stuffing of a saddle is apt to get lumpy sometimes
and rub the horse's back, so in order to minimise the
danger of this happening it is a good thing to beat the
stuffing with your riding stick to keep it spread evenly.

STABLES

Ventilation. It is essential that stables, whether of
the most modern type or converted barns and cattle sheds,
should be well ventilated if horses are to be kept in hard
condition and free from colds and other diseases. Horses

kept in warm and stuffy stables often give the appearance of looking well and sleek in their coats and it is
for this reason that people—especially grooms—are
tempted to exclude as much air as possible.

This is obviously wrong: we ourselves would not
feel our best in the morning if we slept in a fuggy bed-
room; better by far to be warmly covered and have
plenty of air.

It is the same with horses: plenty of air without
draughts is the ideal to be sought when building or
improving existing boxes or again converting farm
buildings into stables. The elimination of draught is
most important as nothing tends to fill the stables with
coughing horses quicker than bad ventilation.

The best type of window is that which when open
has an upward and inward slant, thus forcing the air
over the horse's back.

Apart from windows there are additional methods of
ensuring good ventilation which can be adopted by
consulting any good practical builder. Doors are always
better for being in two horizontal halves and in a row
of outside boxes should as nearly as possible face south.

It is hardly necessary to say that boxes are preferable
to stalls, as horses can walk about or lie down more
easily.

Outside boxes are healthier than those encased in a
building as they get more air and sun, making coughs
and colds less easily spread.

Horses like company, so the isolated box is not to be
recommended.

During the summer months when the horses are
probably out at grass it is an excellent idea to paint or
spray the inside of the boxes with whitewash impreg-
nated with D.D.T., which mixture can be bought from
most chemists.

Roof. As to the roof—apart from slates and tiles—

there are now so many forms of patent composite roofing that it is difficult to give any useful advice on this particular subject but from experience it has been found that thatch has the advantage of being cool in summer and warm in winter, whereas corrugated iron is the very reverse.

Mangers, etc. There would appear to be no point in feeding a horse on, or near, the ground where dirt can collect more easily and where the horse can tread in it; better the old-fashioned manger away from the stable floor and the hay rack not so high that the hay seeds fall into the horse's eyes and ears. A hay net is a good substitute for a rack.

If some sort of gadget can be devised by which the bucket of water can be fixed into a corner of the box without being overturned, it is well worth doing and can be made by any blacksmith.

Drainage. Stables should be well drained or you can have no drains at all. This sounds contradictory, but the explanation will be found when the different types of bedding are discussed. If you have a drainage system there is nothing to beat the ordinary herring-bone form, leading down a slight grade to an open shallow gutter, all of which can easily be swept out.

The squared brick type of floor is more difficult to keep clean.

General Lay-out. It is a great saving of time and labour if the forage can be kept near the stables and incidentally a saving of money if the oats, etc., are kept in dirt and rat-proof bins.

If the stables are situated near to a hot water supply this will be found to be a great blessing.

Bedding. Bedding of some description is necessary in order to induce a horse to lie down and rest his limbs, and the more within reason the better as a scanty bed only leads to injuries such as capped elbows and hocks.

There are different forms of bedding; straw, peat moss litter, sawdust or a combination of these.

There are also different sorts of straw.

Wheat Straw undoubtedly makes the best bed, and owing to the fact that so much more land has come under the plough of late years it is not now very expensive.

Oat Straw is not recommended as horses are inclined to eat it.

Barley Straw is worse still, as if horses do eat it, it may cause colic, also the awns (or beard) are very irritating to the skin. Assuming then that only *Wheat Straw* should be used the method of dealing with it must be considered.

The horse's box should be cleaned out first thing in the morning.

"Mucking out"—as it is more expressively called, consists of removing all the droppings and damp dirty straw and putting it on a manure heap. The comparatively unsoiled straw can then be taken out of the box and if fine dried outside or if necessary in a spare box or somewhere under cover. It may, of course, be necessary to leave it piled up in a corner of the box (away from the manger) but this should be avoided if possible. As the object of giving a horse a good bed is to induce it to lie down, it is as well to put down the new bed before his feed in the middle of the day so that he can have his afternoon's rest, or it may be put down in the evening.

The new straw can then be mixed up with what was left of the old bed—after "mucking out" and well tossed up so that the straws lie across each other and not all in the same direction.

It will be a saving of bedding if droppings are removed from time to time so that they don't have a chance to be trodden in.

Peat Moss Litter makes a good bed and is economical. A good thick bed, five or six inches deep, is necessary.

All droppings and wet litter should be removed constantly until such time as the bedding begins to wear thin when the box should be cleaned out and a new lot put down. This is hard work as it gets congested and heavy. A damp bed of peat moss litter is injurious to the horn of the horse's feet.

A disadvantage of peat moss is that unless precautions are taken it is apt to block the drains.

Sawdust can be used in the same way as peat moss litter—it is, however, cleaner and warmer and requires just as much if not more attention as if left to get damp and mushy it is apt to get hot and maggoty.

The Combination or Continental Type of Bedding. This has advantages over the other kinds of bedding we are used to seeing in this country; firstly it is warm and therefore horses will be found to lie down more often, and secondly, it is labour saving.

Peat Moss Litter is put down first as mentioned before about six inches deep. A generous bed of straw is put on top. Apart from removing the actual droppings at frequent intervals, no "mucking out" has to be done, but instead a new lot of straw if sprinkled on top of the old. It is, of course, not necessary to have a foundation of peat moss—it can be all straw. Sawdust, too, can be tried as a basis for the bed though it might get overheated and maggoty.

Naturally the floor increases in height as the months go by and the time will come when the horse is in danger of hitting its head; then is the time to clean it out and start again—a day's hard work, but, like Christmas, it only comes about once a year.

Captain Humphrey Dixon—the illustrator of this book—has given this type of bedding a very thorough trial, both in Italy in the war and for many years in England, and has found it to work admirably.

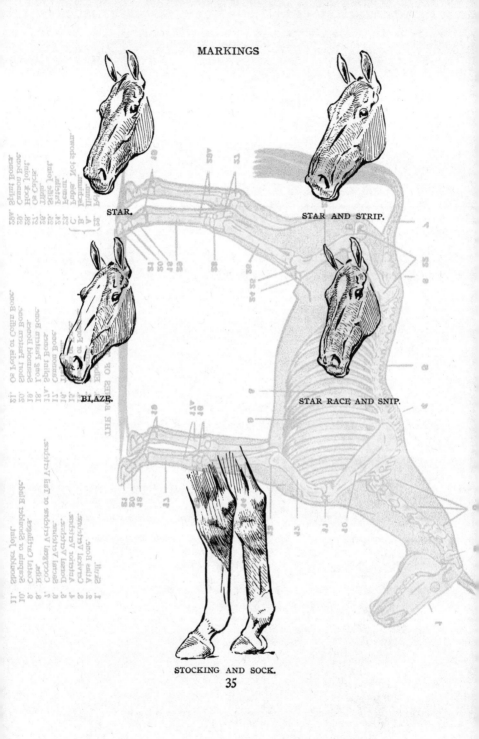

STAR.

STAR AND STRIP.

BLAZE.

STAR RACE AND SNIP.

STOCKING AND SOCK.

35

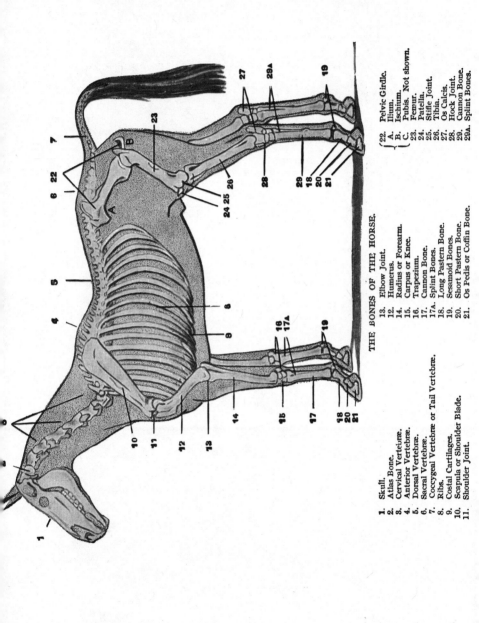

THE BONES OF THE HORSE.

1. Skull.
2. Atlas Bone.
3. Cervical Vertebræ.
4. Anterior Vertebræ.
5. Dorsal Vertebræ.
6. Sacral Vertebræ.
7. Coccygeal Vertebræ or Tail Vertebræ.
8. Ribs.
9. Costal Cartilages.
10. Scapula or Shoulder Blade.
11. Shoulder Joint.
12. Humerus.
13. Elbow Joint.
14. Radius or Forearm.
15. Carpus or Knee.
16. Trapezium.
17. Cannon Bone.
17A. Splint Bones.
18. Long Pastern Bone.
19. Sesamoid Bones.
20. Short Pastern Bone.
21. Os Pedis or Coffin Bone.
22. Pelvic Girdle.
A. Ilium.
B. Ischium.
C. Pubis. Not shown.
23. Femur.
24. Patella.
25. Stifle Joint.
26. Tibia.
27. Os Calcis.
28. Hock Joint.
29. Cannon Bone.
29A. Splint Bones.

CHAPTER II

LAMENESS

IT is not always an easy matter to locate lameness or even to tell which leg is the cause of the trouble.

The horse should first be examined in the stable, and the box should be entered quietly so as to disturb him as little as possible.

A sound horse frequently rests one hind leg, but normally has his weight distributed equally on both forelegs, except in the case of a very tired horse, when he may rest the alternate foreleg as well.

In slight lameness the horse may be standing level, but the pastern of the lame leg will be slightly straighter than that of the sound leg. He may point one foreleg, and in this case it should be noticed whether the heel or the toe is taking the weight of the leg.

A horse generally rests the toe in cases of laminitis or ringbone, and the heel in cases of navicular disease.

If the lameness be in the shoulder, the lame leg appears to hang down and may be slightly behind the other foreleg.

This first glance in the stable may give a clue in case of obscure lameness.

The hand should then be run down each leg in turn with the fingers on the tendons.

By comparing the legs in this way any excessive heat, swelling or tenderness should be discovered.

It is only by constant practice that slight heat in a leg can be detected, and the owner is advised to make a regular habit of running his hand down a horse's leg.

In the same way each foot should be compared, as a hot foot is an indication of injury or disease.

TROTTING A HORSE LAME IN THE OFF FORE.

LAME ON THE NEAR HIND. THE OFF QUARTER DROPPING.

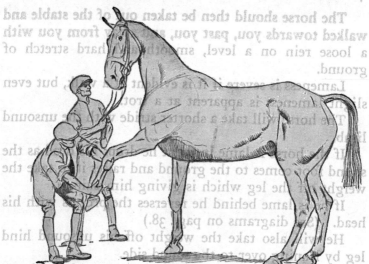

TESTS FOR—SHOULDER LAMENESS.

The horse should then be taken out of the stable and walked towards you, past you, and away from you with a loose rein on a level, smooth and hard stretch of ground.

Lameness is severe if it is evident at a walk, but even slight lameness is apparent at a trot.

The horse will take a shorter stride with the unsound limb.

If the horse is lame in front he drops his head as the sound foot comes to the ground and raises it to take the weight off the leg which is giving him pain.

If he is lame behind he reverses the process with his head. (See diagrams on page 38.)

He will also take the weight off his unsound hind leg by leaning over to the sound side.

Lameness behind is also more apparent when a horse is being turned on the forehand, and this is particularly the case in spavin and stringhalt. Lameness may be more severe if the hock be held flexed and the horse is then trotted (see Spavin lameness).

Sometimes in shoulder lameness he will swing the lame leg slightly or catch his toe on the ground, but the following tests should place the matter beyond doubt.

Tests for Shoulder Lameness. To find out if the pain is in the shoulder pull the horse's leg forwards and then backwards as far as it will go two or three times, and if he flinches or is inclined to rear up, he is probably feeling some pain, and if you have him trotted directly after this treatment he will probably go lamer than before. Some horses are inclined to resent this manipulation, so both shoulders should be tested. (See diagrams on page 39.) A further test for shoulder lameness is to trot the horse uphill and down. If lame in the shoulder, he will be more lame going uphill than down. (N.B.— In the case of foot lameness the reverse is the case.)

In the case of stifle lameness he will bend the stifle hock and fetlock as little as possible.

If a horse is made to rein back he may drag the toe of the leg on which he is lame.

Lameness does not improve with exercise in cases of splints, sore shins, corns, laminitis and sprains.

Veterinary surgeons, by injecting a local anæsthetic, render the leg below the injection insensitive to pain, and so are able to tell whether the seat of lameness lies above or below the point of injection.

When a horse is being examined for soundness, he should be galloped and then tied up in the stable for half an hour to cool down. He should then be brought out again and trotted up, when occult lameness, if present, will be revealed.

Nail Binding is caused by a nail or nails being driven by the farrier too close to the sensitive laminæ of the foot.

Symptoms. The symptoms are pain and lameness, and heat in the foot.

Treatment. Remove the shoe and apply hot antiseptic poultices * for two or three days.

A Pricked Sole is caused by the farrier driving a nail into the sensitive part of the sole, or by a picked-up nail.

Symptoms. Either of these will cause lameness which increases in intensity, and there will be heat and pain in the foot. If the injury is due to shoeing it is probably bad workmanship on the part of the farrier, though there may be a little excuse for him if the horn of the hoof is very thin. Badly shaped nails will make pricking easier, as will the horse himself if he is fidgety and moves at the critical moment when the nail is being driven in.

Treatment. Remove shoe at once.

* See Appendix, page 136.

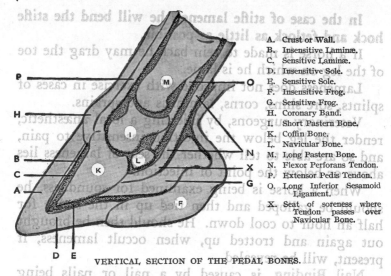

A. Crust or Wall.
B. Insensitive Laminæ.
C. Sensitive Laminæ.
D. Insensitive Sole.
E. Sensitive Sole.
F. Insensitive Frog.
G. Sensitive Frog.
H. Coronary Band.
I. Short Pastern Bone.
K. Coffin Bone.
L. Navicular Bone.
M. Long Pastern Bone.
N. Flexor Perforans Tendon.
P. Extensor Pedis Tendon.
O. Long Inferior Sesamoid Ligament.
X. Seat of soreness where Tendon passes over Navicular Bone.

VERTICAL SECTION OF THE PEDAL BONES.

Have the puncture pared out well to allow good drainage.

Pour iodine into the hole.

Apply antiseptic poultices * twice daily. When the horse trots sound, put on the shoe and place tow soaked in Lysol over the seat of the injury. The tow must be kept in place with a strip of hoop iron wedged under the shoe.

Have anti-tetanus injection given as soon as damage is discovered.

Bruised Sole. The result of a bruised sole is tenderness and possibly extreme lameness. It is caused by the horse treading heavily on a sharp stone, a stub, or by a badly fitted shoe. Any of the above may inflict injury on the sensitive sole of the foot, which the outer wall and sole is inadequate to protect.

Symptoms. The symptoms are heat and pain in the foot, causing lameness. Pressure on the sole with a pair of pincers will cause the horse to flinch.

* See Appendix, page 136.

Treatment. The first thing to do is to remove the shoe and reduce inflammation, which can best be done by means of hot antiseptic poultices.* The poultice should be renewed once or twice a day until all the inflammation and soreness have gone. A laxative diet * is essential. The horse should be carefully re-shod with a light, wide, flat seated out shoe.

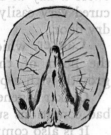

SEAT OF CORN.

A Corn. The cause of a corn in a horse is the same as in a human being. It is undue pressure by the shoe on the seat of injury due to bad shoeing, or to the fact that the shoes have been left on too long. A corn is really a bruise of the sensitive sole in the angle formed by the bar and the wall. Horses that are permanently unshod hardly ever suffer from corns.

The reason why corns appear always in this particular part of the sole is that the horn is thinner in that part.

Treatment. Remove the shoe, pare out the corn to remove pressure, and if pus is found apply antiseptic poultices.* Shoe with a three-quarter shoe.

Thrush is an inflammation of the sensitive frog and the symptoms are rather like those of canker, but it is found in the cleft of the frog only.

It is often a chronic complaint and if neglected at the onset is likely to become serious.

It is more commonly found in the hind feet than in the front.

Cause. It is chiefly found in horses that have been standing in badly drained stables which have not been "mucked out" for some time. It is therefore avoidable.

Symptoms. There may or may not be lameness.

As in canker the presence of thrush is easily detected by the foul smell which accompanies it. The horn in

* See Appendix, pages 136, 141.

the cleft of the frog is soft and spongy, and a thick evil-smelling discharge comes from it.

Treatment. Wash the foot thoroughly with disinfectant solution. Pare out the frog—apply antiseptics such as Stockholm tar and salt in the cavity with a wad of tow to keep the dressing in place. Renew the dressing twice a day at first. Thrush, if taken in time, can be cured very easily. The patient should stand on a clean dry floor.

Canker, which nowadays is rare, is a softening of the horn of the hoof forming a moist cheese-like growth with a particularly objectionable smell.

Canker is generally found where horses are kept under bad conditions such as badly drained stables.

It is also commonly found in marshy districts.

Symptoms. It generally starts in the frog, extending to the sole, and the horn becomes sodden with a moist growth which in time can be squeezed out at the sole.

Sometimes there is considerable pain and lameness, especially when the disease attacks the wall of the foot. The discharge has a foul smell.

Treatment. Remove any loose horn and apply a caustic, such as zinc sulphate, then exert pressure on the affected part by means of a piece of plate or tin placed under the shoe. The disease is often of long duration, which can only be shortened by operation. This is a matter for the veterinary surgeon.

Seedy Toe is an affection of the foot in which the middle layer of horn becomes separated from the sensitive layer underneath. In the space so formed a soft mealy kind of horn is formed. As the name suggests, this is most often found in the toe, but it may occur at any part of the wall of the foot, and starting from the ground runs upwards, sometimes as far as the coronet.

The cause is not always easy to determine, but as the

complaint is brought about by
excessive pressure on the wall of
the foot, then suspicion falls on
the blacksmith, as either a too
tightly hammered toe clip or a
too tightly driven nail will cause
the trouble.

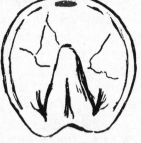

SEEDY TOE

It may also occur after laminitis.

Symptoms. The blacksmith
will generally be the first to detect the presence of seedy
toe when he is using his hammer, as a knock with it
will produce a hollow sound, and driving a nail into the
seedy toe area is like knocking a nail into a thin wall
when it goes into space. The horse will go lame when
the affected area is large, but not when it is first
beginning.

Treatment. Pare away the seedy formation, dress with
tar and tow, and put on a shoe which has no bearing on
the damaged tissue.

Blister the coronet to stimulate a new growth of
horn.

In very bad cases an operation consisting in cutting
away the wall right up to the seat of the trouble is
necessary to effect a permanent cure.

Contracted Heels. The blacksmith is sometimes to
blame, as if the frog is pared away too much it becomes
dry and contracted, and thus does not come in contact
with the ground and encourage the expansion of the
heel.

Similarly, undue cutting away of the bars will allow
the heels to grow inwards. Calkins which take all the
weight off the frog allow the latter to contract with the
same result. A contracted foot is in all cases dangerous
as it is a contributory cause of navicular disease.

Symptoms. The walls of the foot are contracted in

one or more places in the regions of the quarters and heels and on one or both sides of the foot. This condition must not be confounded with "odd feet," in which one foot, though of good shape, may be smaller than its fellow. Odd feet are often hereditary or due to some injury as a foal or yearling which causes unequal distribution of weight for a period.

Some horses are born with contracted feet. In the case of a horse which has been lame for some time, the foot of the lame leg may become contracted, owing to its having borne less weight than its fellow.

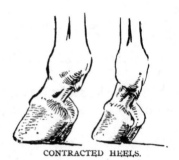

CONTRACTED HEELS.

Treatment. Frog pressure is both the prevention and cure of this ailment.

The sole should be well rasped down at the heels, so that the frog makes contact with the ground, which will encourage its expansion.

In severe cases a run at grass should be given and the horse shod with tips.*

In extreme cases grooving of the wall of the hoof may be necessary.

Brittle Feet. These are due to a dry condition of the horn.

Sea water and sand are thought to be a predisposing cause.

* See Appendix, pages 145, 146.

Treatment. Keep water away from the feet.

Stimulate the coronet to produce new horn by means of a red blister.*

Dress the horn two or three times a day with castor oil.

Keratoma (*Horn Tumour*). This is a horny growth on the interior wall of the horn of the hoof. It is due to an excessive activity of the horn-producing laminæ which may follow an injury or be caused by the presence of irritant matter in the foot. It is usually present near the toe.

Symptoms. These tumours are not easy to detect in

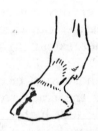 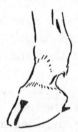

CLASP TO PREVENT SAND   SAND CRACK.
CRACK SPREADING.

the early stages, but if the sole be pared the white line of health between the sole and the horn will be seen to curve inwards below the tumour.

Inflammation and lameness may be present, and a fistula may form which will discharge pus.

Treatment. All pressure must be removed from the area concerned and veterinary aid called in.

Sand Crack is a crack in the wall of the hoof running downwards from the coronet to the ground, or sometimes only a part of the way down. The horse may or may not go lame.

The crack is in many cases not visible near the

* See Appendix, page 139.

coronet, but owing to pressure it spreads as it is growing out. Sand crack is therefore generally noticed near the sole, as shown in the illustration.

Cause. A tread on the inside of the coronet or an injury to the coronary band. It is also caused by rasping away the outside wall of the foot so that the natural secretion which keeps the hoof moist is lost, the horn then becoming dry, hard and brittle.

Treatment. Remove all pressure from the crack.

If at the toe, shoe with quarter clips.*

A clasp may be put across the crack.

Blister the coronet, thus stimulating a growth of new horn.

The crack may be isolated by making a groove with a hot iron, which any capable farrier can execute. Its object is that the crack shall not extend to the new horn.

If a sand crack suppurates, the horn must be cut away to allow the pus to escape and the crack treated by standing the foot in an antiseptic foot bath.

False Quarter is a horizontal crack in the hoof and is caused by an injury to the coronet. The secretion of horn is checked.

Treatment. New horn formation is encouraged by the application of a red blister to the coronet.

Quittor is the name given to a fistulous sore on the coronet. A quittor comes from one of the following causes:—

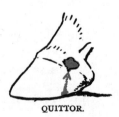

QUITTOR.

(1) From a blow of some sort such as a tread—i.e., when a horse, coming on behind, treads on the coronet of the horse in front; or an over-reach—i.e., when a horse strikes his foreleg with the inside of his hind shoe in galloping or jumping.

* See Appendix, page 144.

(2) From pus working upwards from a suppurating corn.

(3) From a suppurating sand crack.

(4) From a picked-up nail which has been neglected.

Symptoms. There will be a good deal of pain and consequent lameness, and later a discharge.

Treatment. Apply an antiseptic poultice * and send for a veterinary surgeon.

Laminitis is an inflammation of the sensitive laminæ which are directly under the horny wall of the foot. It is a very serious disease and is also most painful as can be imagined when one considers that there is no room for expansion under the hard, unrelenting horn of the hoof.

It is more common in front than behind.

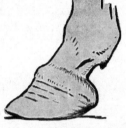

THE CONCAVE AND RINGED APPEARANCE OF THE FOOT FOLLOWING ACUTE LAMINITIS.

Causes. (1) Being made to do hard work when in an unfit condition or galloping about when turned out to grass when the ground is hard.

(2) Flat feet are most prone to this disease.

(3) Too much heating food, such as oats, barley, wheat, peas or beans, and not enough exercise.

(4) Too much weight being placed on one foot—e.g., if the other is injured, especially if the horse has not been put on a laxative diet. For the same reason top-heavy stallions or mares in foal are prone to this disease, especially if they are indiscreetly fed.

(5) After a bad attack of colic.

(6) After foaling.

Symptoms. Inflammation accompanied by abnormal heat and pain. A horse suffering from laminitis will resent being asked to move about, and when it does will

* See Appendix, page 136.

do so on its heels with its back arched and its four feet kept together as much as possible—in fact it may show every symptom of acute pain, such as sweating and groaning. Anybody who has had blood poisoning under a finger nail or toe nail will be able to realise what a horse has to endure with laminitis. No wonder, then, that when it once gets down and finds a little relief from getting the weight off the foot or feet it is, to put it mildly, reluctant to get up again. Its temperature* may be anything from 103° to 106°.

Treatment. Give a physic ball.* Put him on bran mashes. Apply bran poultices* to the fore feet and give plenty of bedding to encourage the horse to lie down.

Opinions differ as to whether the shoes should be removed or not.

Send for a veterinary surgeon, as in some cases injections of adrenalin are advisable.

Navicular Disease is one of the most serious diseases that a horse can have, and is unfortunately only too common. "Serious" is perhaps a mild term to use since it might almost be described as fatal, because, there being no known permanent cure, sooner or later the sufferer, for humanitarian reasons, has to be put down. Briefly, it is a corrosive ulcer on the navicular bone, and is practically confined to the fore feet. It is seen mostly in horses doing fast work.

Cause. (1) Concussion, i.e., too much fast or strenuous work, especially after a long rest.

(2) Contracted heels.

(3) Short, upright pasterns are more prone to navicular than are long, sloping ones.

(4) Any type of shoe with high heels if worn constantly is apt to cause navicular, no pressure being taken by the frog as Nature intended.

* See Appendix, pages 141, 136.

(5) It may be hereditary.

Symptoms. It is gradual in its onset and insidious in its appearance. The first sign is a pointing of a fore foot in the stable or each fore foot alternately. Some horses will always point a fore foot in the stable to rest themselves, which fact may be misleading, but if they do not rest the alternate hind leg at the same time disease such as navicular must be suspected.

The next symptom to appear is lameness when the horse goes out, which may wear off with exercise or in soft going. There will, however, be heat in the foot after a long journey.

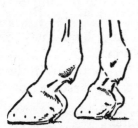 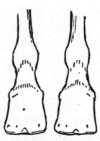

THE SHAPE OF THE FEET DUE TO NAVICULAR DISEASE.

In the course of time the horse will become more lame and pottery in his gait and will be inclined to stumble. In the end he will become so bad as to be unworkable.

In appearance, the foot will generally become contracted at the heels and the sole concave in appearance.

Treatment. There is no cure. Once its presence has been definitely diagnosed by a veterinary surgeon it is far better to have the horse destroyed as any treatment can only be of a temporary nature. It is cruel to work a horse with this disease and also dangerous to the rider.

Palliative treatment, i.e., the application of cold swabs consists of tying a piece of sacking round the coronet loosely and keeping it wet with cold water. If the horse be kept on a clay bed * it will relieve the pain and may prolong his period of usefulness.

It is not intended to recommend the operation of unnerving in these notes since in no case can it be described as "treatment."

A Ring-bone is a bony enlargement round the top of the hoof when it is called "low ring-bone," or round the pastern bones—in which case it is called "high ring-bone."

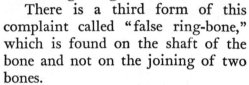

There is a third form of this complaint called "false ring-bone," which is found on the shaft of the bone and not on the joining of two bones.

Cause. (1) Ring-bone may quite likely be hereditary.

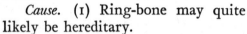

RING-BONE.

(2) It is also common in horses whose pasterns are too straight, on account of the exaggerated jar on the bone.

(3) A blow may cause ring-bone.

(4) Shoes not being removed regularly, thus allowing the heels to grow too long. Frog pressure is removed and the jar on the feet increased.

Symptoms. The first symptoms of ring-bone are rather difficult to determine—the horse may come out slightly lame in the morning, and this lameness will be persistent. The difficulty of tracing the lameness to ring-bone is increased by the fact that there is no heat to be felt, practically no pain and nothing to show in the way of a swelling.

After a week or two heat will be felt, and the horse appears to be in pain.

In the case of advanced high ring-bone the bony growth can be felt, but in the low variety there is no

* See Appendix, page 138.

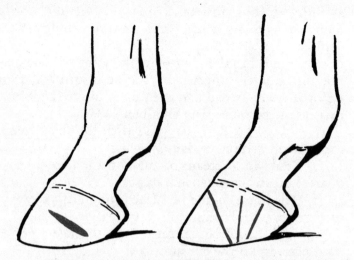

TWO METHODS OF GROOVING FREQUENTLY USED FOR SIDE BONE
AND OTHER FOOT DISEASES.

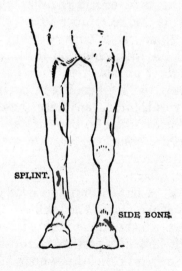

SPLINT.

SIDE BONE.

53

swelling to show for some time; in fact, not until the hoof changes its shape and becomes bulgy at the coronet.

Although in false ring-bone the joint of the bones is not immediately affected by the bony growth, it may unfortunately extend and eventually affect the joint. In this case it becomes true ring-bone.

Treatment. (1) Rest the horse with the shoes removed and put on a laxative diet.

(2) Stand in a stream or turn on the hose-pipe for a quarter of an hour twice a day.

(3) The horse should be turned rough in a straw yard or big box with bedding of peat moss or sawdust.

(4) Feet should be trimmed so as to have a perfectly level bearing on the surface.

(5) Blister, but consult your veterinary surgeon before doing so, as it may possibly do more harm than good, added to which he may recommend point firing or opening the foot as an alternative.

Unnerving is a drastic remedy which is sometimes adopted but is not recommended.

A Side Bone is a bony growth on either lateral cartilage of the foot, common in heavy horses and also found in lighter breeds.

Cause. (1) Possibly hereditary, or it may come from a blow or tread, but in any case there is a natural tendency for the cartilage to become ossified where it joins on to the pedal bone.

(2) Narrow feet.

(3) High calkins.

Symptoms. A hard lump and heat can be felt on the coronet on either side of the heel.

Treatment. If the horse is not lame no treatment is necessary. If lameness persists he must be rested and the veterinary surgeon called in, who will have to resort to blistering, firing or, in very bad cases, to grooving the wall of the foot to relieve the pressure of the ossified cartilage.

A Split Pastern. This condition can sometimes only be established definitely by means of X-ray, but is sure to be accompanied by extreme lameness.

It is believed by some authorities to be caused by the tendons contracting simultaneously instead of alternately. It does not necessarily occur at fast paces.

Fractures occur more frequently in the short than in the long pastern.

Treatment. Send for a veterinary surgeon. Unless the fracture is a bad one, slings are unnecessary ; it is more usual to rely on Plaster of Paris.* A soft bed of sawdust is essential.

Sessamoiditis is an inflammation of the bones situated just above and behind the fetlock joint.

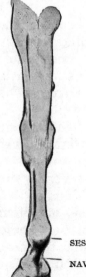

Cause. Faulty conformation, such as upright pasterns or turned out toes, the latter causing the horse to go close at the fetlocks.

Symptoms. The horse will be lame on and off and heat in the fetlock joint will vary from day to day.

There may or may not be a swelling in the fetlock joint, and in bad cases the horse will not bring the heel of the shoe on to the ground.

Treatment. Rest and blister or pin-fire. There is no certain cure.

SESSAMOIDITIS.

NAVICULAR.

Swollen Legs. In horses

* See Appendix, page 139.

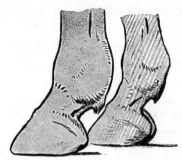

SWOLLEN FETLOCKS. THE RESULT
OF SPRAIN OR WEAR.

which have done a considerable amount of work the legs will frequently be found to be puffy after standing in the stable.

This is due to wear and the congestion of blood in the limbs.

In order to check the congestion the legs should be hand-rubbed upwards towards the heart and pressure bandages should be applied.

Pressure bandages should have plenty of cotton wadding next the skin, retained in position by fairly tight wool or crêpe bandages. They should extend from below the knee over the pastern to the coronet.

An alternative treatment which has been used with success is 2 lb. of blue clay, 4 tablespoonfuls of methylated spirits, 4 tablespoonfuls of vinegar, 1 tablespoonful of glycerine. Sufficient soft water is added to mix the whole into a soft paste, which is spread on the leg after work with a flat piece of wood. This should be re-applied as it flakes off.

Sprains. The position and names of the various tendons and ligaments will be found in the accompanying illustration.

Sprains generally occur in the forelegs but occasionally in the hind.

Sprains do not often occur without warning. As a rule, there is slight heat due to strain, which has passed unnoticed and the actual sprain takes place when the horse is worked in this condition.

Cause. A sprain may be caused in any of the following ways:—

(1) By pulling the horse up suddenly as in polo.

(2) By all the weight of the body falling on one leg.

(3) By too much galloping as when training for a race.

(4) By galloping or jumping when the going is heavy or holding. This is more likely to happen if the horse is unfit or tired.

(5) By leaving the toes too long.

(6) Through defective conformation, such as long, sloping pasterns, a crooked leg or legs that are tied below the knee.

(7) Through ring-bone or enlarged pasterns which hinder or restrict the free movement of the joints and which mechanically cause the relaxation of the tendons.

(8) By slipping or getting cast in the stable; though this is very rare.

Symptoms. There is a good deal of pain when the perforatus and its check ligament are affected—but not so much when the suspensory ligament is strained.

There will be pain, swelling and heat in the tendon.

When one division only of the suspensory ligament is strained the horse may not be lame

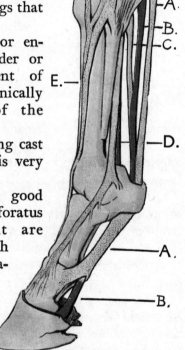

A. Perforatus tendon.
B. Perforans tendon.
C. Check ligament.
D. Suspensory ligament.
E. Extensor tendon.

for some hours after the strain has occurred; for instance, a horse may contract the injury during the course of a race or a hunt; it is only when action has ceased and muscular re-contraction occurs that the inability will be apparent.

The best means of diagnosing the seat of strain is to hold up the leg and press the various tendons with the fingers and thumb until the horse flinches.

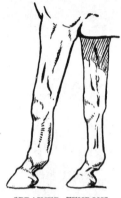

Treatment. Treatment will depend on the gravity of the case, but rest is always essential.

In the case of mild sprain, resulting in heat but not appreciable swelling, cold-water bandages * or cooling lotion will be all that is necessary. Generally, however, the matter is more serious than this. There will be considerable inflammation and tenderness, which must be removed by means of hot fomentations * or Anti-phlogistine applied hot and left on for forty-eight hours.

SPRAINED TENDONS.

A high-heeled shoe will give relief.

In extreme cases blistering or firing must be resorted to, and the horse given a long rest. A recurrence of the trouble under strain, such as fast work, jumping, etc., is frequently to be expected.

A Splint is a bony enlargement on the cannon bone or splint bones, generally on the inside of the fore limbs, but sometimes on the outside as well. It is seldom seen in the hind limbs. They most often appear in young horses and are seldom thrown out after a horse is six years old, except as the result of a blow. For illustration, see p. 53. It is rare for a horse that has done any work at all at six years old not to have splints, and too much

* See Appendix, pages 137, 139.

importance should not be attached to them unless they are so placed that they interfere with the use of a tendon or ligament, or are causing lameness.

Splints are generally caused by the horse's legs being jarred unnecessarily when he is still young—such as jumping on to a hard surface or trotting fast on the road.

They may also arise from bad conformation of the legs and feet; or, again, from too much pressure being brought to bear on the outside of the foot by faulty shoeing.

Symptoms. A splint in its early conception is an insidious complaint: it arrives without any warning. There is often nothing to be felt and yet the horse is lame—and the lameness increases with exercise. The horse may walk sound and yet trot quite lame; on the other hand, if the horse is given no work he may trot sound for a little way and then go lame—all of which is perplexing. Splints, once they are set, rarely cause lameness unless they are in a position which interferes with the tendons or ligaments.

The worst position for a splint is high up and under the knee. This is called a knee splint. If it is well to the front it will not be troublesome for long.

If the splint is on a hind leg the horse will rarely go lame.

The best way, however, to find a splint when it first starts is to pick up the foot and press your fingers down the splint bone until the horse flinches, remembering always that some horses are more sensitive than others.

Treatment. At the outset cold-water bandages or cooling lotion * will probably be all that is required, but in persistent cases blistering or pin-firing must be resorted to. The horse should be given such work as

* See Appendix, page 138.

he is capable of doing, e.g., if he walks sound, let him have walking exercise.

Sore Shins. This is an inflammation of the membrane covering the front of the cannon bone, the front tendon being thereby extended.

Cause. It is due to galloping on hard ground, and occurs most frequently in young racehorses.

Symptoms. There will be heat and swelling of the membrane covering the cannon bone. It may or may not cause lameness.

Treatment. In mild cases massage and rest are advisable. Diluted tincture of arnica (4 tablespoonfuls to 1 pint of water) dabbed on with cotton wool at frequent intervals will ease the pain.

In bad cases it may be necessary to apply a mild blister.

Loss of form in a young racehorse may well be due to a sore shin.

Windgalls are swellings just above the fetlock and on either side of it. Though unsightly, they will not cause lameness, and, unlike thorough-pins, are, if small, not a technical unsoundness.

They are caused by strain and hard work.

Treatment. Treat as for thorough-pin. Such drastic measures as blistering, etc., are hardly worth while except for show purposes since the condition does not affect the usefulness of the horse. By raising the heels with calkins * the strain may be alleviated.

Bandages in the stable are useful but once used they must not be discontinued.

Thorough-pin or Through Pin. *Symptoms.* A distension of the tendon-sheath immediately above and on either side of the point of the hock. It amounts to a technical unsoundness, though it seldom causes lameness.

* See Appendix, pages 143, 144.

Treatment. If the thorough-pin is small no treatment is necessary and work can continue, but if large rest the horse and apply iodine ointment or better still a blister which should be repeated every six weeks until the swelling gets smaller or disappears.

A Curb is not such a serious affair as it is generally considered to be. Once successfully treated it will probably cause no further trouble from a practical point of view. It is, however, unsightly, and must be counted as a weakness and therefore detracts from the value of the horse.

The cause is difficult to fix exactly, but it can invariably be attributed to undue strain, e.g., when a horse has jumped badly, possibly out of a sticky take-off.

Horses with sickle hocks are more liable to curbs than others, especially if they are excitable and fidgety.

Young cart horses are very likely to throw out curbs when too heavy a load is put behind them.

Symptoms. A horse with a curb is not necessarily lame. If he does go lame he goes on his toe, and when standing still he will raise the heel off the ground.

Curb results in a thickening of the tendon or ligament on the back of the hock—about a hand's breadth below the point.

False curb is seen when the head of the metatarsal bone is unduly large, and viewed from the side gives the effect of "true curb." False curb is not an unsoundness.

H H.O.   E

THROUGH-PIN.

WINDGALLS.

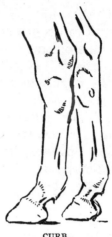

CURB.

Treatment. Rest the heel with calkins or a wedge-shaped shoe, and apply plenty of cold water; then if necessary apply a blister or such preparations as Iodine Ointment, Radiol or Reducine, which should be rubbed in thoroughly for several days (not, however, after the skin begins to crack). After the skin has peeled off the process may be repeated if necessary.

Firing, while unsightly, will seldom fail to effect a permanent cure and is to be recommended in all severe cases otherwise a recurrence of lameness will probably result when work starts again.

Bog Spavin is a chronic, puffy swelling on the inside and a little to the front of the hock, but it cannot be counted amongst the more serious diseases.

Symptoms. In most cases the horse is not even lame.

Small bulges may be seen on the inside of the hock.

If a horse does go lame on a bog spavin there is no doubt about the matter as he carries his leg and swings it clear of the ground.

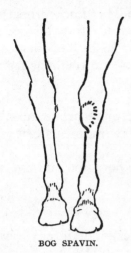
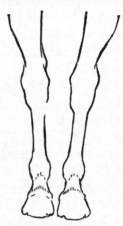

BOG SPAVIN.   BONE SPAVIN.

Bog spavins are most often found in horses with very straight hocks.

They are caused by some strain, such as slipping backwards or from overwork.

As in the case of thorough-pins, bog spavins may be considered in the light of a provision of Nature to protect a badly formed joint.

Treatment. Treatment as for thorough-pin.

A Bone Spavin is a bony growth inside and just below the hock joint, which need not be a serious disease, unless it causes lameness.

Occult spavin, as the name implies, is more difficult to detect and far more serious. The growth occurs between two of the bones of the hock, just below the joint and on the inner side, but no enlargement is noticeable, though the horse will most probably go lame.

Predisposition to this disease is often hereditary. Horses with sickle hocks and cow hocks are susceptible to this complaint. Even with good hocks a bone spavin may occur if undue concussion or strain occurs as in jumping out of deep going.

Symptoms. As he cannot bend his hock properly at the trot, he will shorten his stride, drag his toe and appear to drop his hip at each step as his lame leg comes to the ground. The toe of the shoe on the lame leg will be worn.

Lameness will be more noticeable when the horse first starts to move, and will be more pronounced still if the hock be held flexed for a few moments before the horse is trotted.

In occult spavin the lameness does not improve with exercise.

Treatment. Rest.

Raise the heels of the shoe.

Firing or blistering is quicker than any passive treatment, but many cases are incurable.

Knee Spavin is a bony growth at the back of the knee, on the inner side. It is caused by a blow or by a strain. It is much more serious than hock spavin, but fortunately far less common. It occurs mostly in race-horses.

Knee spavin, unlike spavin of the hock, is not hereditary.

Symptoms. A horse with knee spavin may or may not go lame at first, but there will be a distinct swelling of the knee. He will not be able to bend his knee or put his foot out very far, and to avoid having to try to do these things he will move with a circular sweep of the affected leg, appearing to try to bring the heel of his foot on to the ground before his toe.

He will show signs of pain if the knee is bent by picking up the foot.

Treatment. Blister or fire.

String Halt. It is not known what causes string halt, though there have been many ingenious theories put forward from time to time. One is almost safe. however, in classing it as a nervous disease.

Symptoms. It is a curious disease, in that it causes a horse suddenly to snatch up one or both hind legs when walking, and occasionally when trotting. Sometimes it is hardly noticeable, but in bad cases the horse almost kicks itself in the stomach. It is not often found in horses under five years of age.

The symptoms appear more exaggerated when the horse has been resting or when backed or turned in small circles.

Treatment. There is no treatment that will cure the horse of string halt except an operation, and this is uncertain, but since the affliction detracts little, if at all, from his usefulness, such operation can only be recommended in the case of a valuable show animal.

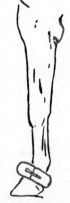

A **Capped Elbow** is nearly always caused either by being bruised by the heel of the shoe when lying down (especially if in a stall), from lack of bedding, or from a rough, uneven floor.

Symptoms. The point of the elbow will probably be bruised and swollen. The horse may not go lame, or if lame will soon become sound again.

CAPPED ELBOW AND SAUSAGE BOOT.

If the swelling is very big, it points to an abscess. If the swelling is hard, the capped elbow is chronic. There will be no heat, pain or lameness unless the bruise is recent.

Treatment. If quite recent, massage with ointment of marsh mallow, iodine ointment or lead lotion. A reducing paste * such as Fuller's earth and vinegar smeared on every day, is very effective.

If an abscess has formed, it must be lanced and syringed out frequently with a solution of iodine (1 part iodine to 12 parts water).

* See Appendix, page 138.

For horses that are liable to cap their elbows a stuffed leather ring (commonly called a sausage boot) strapped round the coronet may prevent a recurrence, but plenty of bedding and a 3/4 shoe is more certain to do so.

A capped elbow which has become hard and callous may be removed by an operation.

A Capped Hock is caused by the horse kicking in the stable, or by a shortage of bedding when the horse lies down.

Symptoms. There are two kinds: (1) involving the

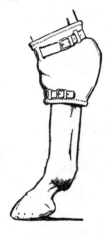

HOCK BOOT.

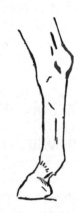

CAPPED HOCK.

synovial bursa, shows a slight swelling on each side of the hock-cap. This may be accompanied by extreme lameness. (2) a less serious form, showing large swelling on the point of the hock. It is unsightly but not serious, and there may be no sign of lameness.

Treatment. Give plenty of bedding in a loose box. If the case is recent put on a paste made of whitening and vinegar or antiphlogistine. If it is callous a blister or a charge will be necessary.

Preventive Treatment. Sufficient bedding and a hock boot.

Stifle Lameness. Watch the horse from behind as he is trotted away and you will notice that he slightly raises his quarter on the side he is lame.

His step will be shorter and altogether he will save his lame leg by only slightly bending his stifle, hock and fetlock.

In addition, the foot of the lame leg follows the track of the opposite fore foot; that is, if the horse is lame on the off stifle the foot follows the track of the near fore foot, and also appears to trot away from the lame side. The toe is not dragged, this being a sign of hock trouble.

Treatment. If the lameness is due to a sprain of the stifle, it should be treated as an ordinary sprain with fomentations, etc.

It may, however, be due to dislocation of the stifle joint, in which case veterinary aid should be called in to get the joint back into position.

Shoulder Lameness. A horse is most likely to strain his shoulder when he slips, lands badly over a jump or falls with his forelegs spread out.

Symptoms. As previously mentioned, in tests for lameness the horse will trot short and resent his foreleg being pulled backward and forward. A slight swelling and heat may possibly be noticeable.

Treatment. Rest is absolutely necessary.

Run cold water over the shoulder with a hose-pipe twice a day for an hour at a time if possible; also massage with a soap liniment. When the first inflammation has subsided, a mild blister applied to the shoulder will expedite the cure.

A Broken Pelvis is not common in horses, but it is possible for a horse to break his pelvis and the fracture be unobserved.

A horse may break his pelvis in many ways: (1) by severe muscular strain, such as slipping on a smooth road, etc.; (2) by a fall on a hard surface; (3) in jumping;

(4) by hitting the sides of a gatepost, narrow doorway, or the like.

Symptoms. The horse will be lame—possibly very lame. It is probable that a creaking noise at 'the seat of the break can be heard, and that there may be a swelling between the legs.

Treatment. Complete rest for many weeks, in slings.

CHAPTER III

INJURIES

Tetanus   is a disease caused by *Bacillus tetani* and is included in this chapter as it is through a wound that this bacillus gains entry to the horse.

This disease is more prevalent in some districts than in others. Death results in nine cases out of ten once the symptoms have developed.

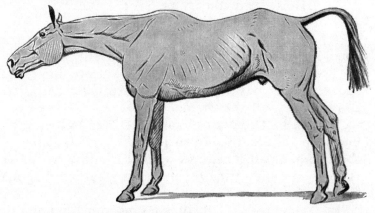

TETANUS.

Symptoms. The temperature rises to between 103° and 105° F.

The first symptom is a general stiffening of the limbs, and the animal will stand with nose and tail stretched out.

The membrane of the eye will extend over the eyeball.

The horse is in a nervous state, and any sudden noise or movement will cause him to tauten every muscle in his body.

69

Later the jaws become set and the horse can only suck nourishment.

Treatment. Send for a veterinary surgeon at once.

Prevention. The modern method is to give the horse an injection of a toxoid which after another injection in a year's time will give a lifelong immunity.

If a horse has not been given toxoid an anti-tetanus serum should be given as early as possible after any deep wound: this will give a temporary immunity only.

Treatment of Wounds. Wounds are divided into three groups:—

    (1) Punctures.

    (2) Cuts and tears.

    (3) Deep wounds.

(1) *Punctures* are dangerous in that they may be very small and consequently are apt to be overlooked.

They may also heal from the surface first, thus enclosing any pus which would eventually necessitate the reopening of the wound.

Treatment. Dress with iodine, and keep well syringed out with mild antiseptic two or three times daily. In the case of small punctures where syringing is impracticable, antiphlogistine or antiseptic poultices * should be applied.

(2) *Cuts or tears.* If there is no inflammation and the wound is clean, leave it alone as much as possible and do not put on a bandage.

Bathe with salt and water (1 in 100) though this is not actually an antiseptic, or any of the antiseptics mentioned in the appendix can be used, but remember most antiseptics delay healing.

(3) *Deep Wounds.* First the bleeding must be stopped. This should not be difficult if the bleeding is only from veins. Blood from veins is dull red. Arterial blood is bright scarlet, and issues in spurts from the wound.

* See Appendix, page 136.

Copious applications of cold water should be sufficient to stop venous bleeding. If a limb artery has been cut a tourniquet applied above it will help to arrest the flow of blood.

If the arterial bleeding is severe the cut should be bathed continuously in cold water and veterinary aid sought at once.

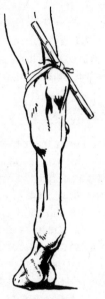

After bleeding has ceased the next object is to get the wound thoroughly clean. This is done with a mild antiseptic syringed into the wound or applied with clean cotton-wool.*

Free drainage to a wound is essential, and to allow this it may be necessary for the wound to be opened up.

The removal of the inflammation comes next, and is best done by means of hot fomentations with a little disinfectant or common salt in the water.* These should be repeated at frequent intervals until all the inflammation has gone and the discharge has completely ceased.

TOURNIQUET.

The wound may then be dressed with salt and water, or a 1 in 40 solution of carbolic acid or perchloride of mercury, strength 1 in 1000.* Antiseptic gauze should be soaked in one of these solutions, packed into the wound, and kept in place with a linen bandage.

The dressing should be changed and the wound syringed out with the same antiseptic twice a day at first and once a day later.

Do not be in a hurry for the wound to heal; if it is kept clean it is sure to heal, and the essential thing is that it should heal from the base outwards.

* See Appendix, page 134.

The box or stall should be kept scrupulously clean and sweet to avoid possible reinfection.

Where tetanus is prevalent an anti-tetanus injection should be given within twelve hours.

In all cases where inflammation is present recovery will be assisted by putting the horse on a low, cooling diet with little or no oats.

If a wound has been septic the skin generally will not unite and the wound becomes filled with grandulated tissue known as proud flesh. It may be necessary to burn this back with caustics such as nitrate of silver.

Wounds near Joints. Especial treatment is needed in the case of wounds near joints owing to the danger of the joint becoming open and joint oil flowing. If a wound near a joint be deep it is advisable to get expert aid and not to allow an inexperienced person to use a probe when searching for foreign matter in the wound.

If there is no fear of an open joint the treatment is the same as for an ordinary wound.

Broken Knees. If the injury to the knee or knees be deep there is grave danger of an open joint, and the horse owner is well advised to call in his veterinary surgeon.

This advice is given as the permanent blemish can be considerably reduced if expert advice is obtained immediately after the mishap.

If the skin is not broken and only the hair is removed no treatment is necessary except perhaps the application of one of the many patent hair-restorers, which may encourage new growth of hair.

If the skin be broken first-aid treatment consists of (1) tying the horse's head up so that he cannot injure the knee; (2) cleaning the wound with warm water to which a little disinfectant is added; (3) dusting an antiseptic powder over the wound and keeping clean.

Saddle and Harness Sores.   As these are caused by
badly fitting saddles and harness, it is obvious, therefore,
that prevention is better than cure, and so particular
care should be taken to see that everything fits correctly
before starting work.

In riding horses this is particularly necessary where
a lady's saddle is concerned, as the saddle has to take
more strain on one side than on the other, and whilst
considering this subject it is as well to remember that,
even though a horse has been ridden regularly in a man's
saddle without injury, the first long work in a lady's
saddle is more than likely to scald the horse's back on
the loins where it has not been hardened by the astride
saddle.

Care should also be taken that horses that are just up
from grass, or for other reasons have not had a saddle
on for some time, should not have one on for more
than an hour or so at a time till the back is hardened.

Girth galls are very troublesome, but should not occur
if care is taken in tightening the girths and seeing that
the girths are kept soft.

Horses in soft condition are particularly liable to
girth galls, but even in hard conditioned horses they will
occur if the skin is pinched or wrinkled under the girth.
To avoid this, the girths must be tightened up level,
and the hand should be passed under the girth in a
downward direction to smooth out any wrinkles in the
skin.

Treatment. If a girth gall occurs substitute a string
girth or put a motor-cycle tube round the girth. Apply
a cooling lotion to the galls and continue work unless
they are severe.

Curb Galls. Too tight a curb chain or one that has
been twisted wrongly is most likely to rub a sore place.
(The curb chain should be twisted from the near side in
a clockwise direction.)

Treatment. The best treatment for all saddle or harness galls is complete rest from the offending saddlery concerned. Wash with disinfectant * diluted in warm water and dress after with boracic powder.

As a prevention, three tablespoonfuls of salt to a pint of water will help to harden the skin, and this should be swabbed on the parts likely to be affected after coming in from work, especially in the cases of young horses with tender skins, or horses that have not had saddle or harness on for some time.

If it is absolutely essential to work a horse with a sore back or withers, the only way to prevent further trouble is to put an old felt nummah under the saddle, which has been cut so as to take pressure off the affected part.

Sitfast. This is a hard, painful swelling on the horse's back.

It may be caused by pressure due to an ill-fitting saddle, or by any continuous pressure on an incompletely healed sore.

Symptoms. A lump will appear and, in the case of an old sore, a hard, dry skin will form over the sore, which will later slough off, leaving the sitfast. This will get larger and more painful the longer it is neglected, and a horse may be laid up for some time.

Treatment. The sitfast must be cut out by a veterinary surgeon, after which it is essential to keep the wound thoroughly clean until healed.

At first iodine may be used, and later the wound should be dabbed frequently with a mixture of 2 table-spoonfuls of powdered alum to 1 pint of water.

Unless the roots of the sitfast are not completely removed it will not heal.

If the original sore had been allowed to heal properly

* See Appendix, page 134.

before the horse was saddled again, no sitfast would
have formed.

Thorn Injuries. The legs of a horse should be well
examined after hunting and all thorns removed, taking
great care not to break off the point of the thorn inside
the flesh, as not only are most thorns poisonous but also
they are inclined to work inwards and may cause serious
trouble in the future especially if near a joint or tendon.

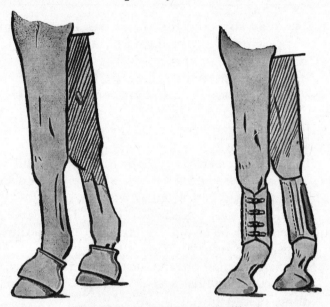

TWO FORMS OF OVER-REACH BOOTS.

If it is suspected that the point of a thorn has
remained embedded antiseptic poultices * should be
applied.

Bruises are contusions of the skin caused by blows,
etc.

In horses they are not always very conspicuous, even
when a considerable amount of blood has coagulated in
the damaged tissues.

* See Appendix, page 136.

Treatment consists of cold fomentations, or, if possible, a stream of cold water directed on the affected part.

After the acute pain has subsided the part should be massaged and vinegar and water or any other cooling lotion * applied. Gentle exercise is advisable at this stage if no lameness is present.

Over-reaches are caused by the inside of the toe of the hind shoe striking the foreleg on the heel or on the back of the coronet.

They may also occur on the fetlock or even higher.

Over-reaches occur during fast paces or when jumping, and more often when the going is deep.

As a general preventive measure the toe of the hind shoes should be bevelled off and the whole shoe set well back.

Horses liable to over-reach must wear over-reach boots when hunting.

Over-reaches vary very much in severity, and when they occur iodine should be applied at once, and in the stable they should be treated as wounds.

Brushing and Speedy Cutting. These are both caused by the hoof of one leg striking the opposite one, thus causing an injury.

Brushing occurs on the inside of the fetlocks (in front or behind), whilst speedy cutting is below and on the inside of the knee.

They generally occur in horses that are poor or weak but may also be caused by bad shoeing. Horses with defective conformation and consequently bad action are very likely to receive these injuries.

Treatment. Treat as a bruise or wound.

If the horse is in bad condition give him light steady work until his strength has been regained.

If a horse in good condition continues to brush or speedy-cut the shoes should be examined.

* See Appendix, page 138.

The shoes must not project at all beyond the wall of the hoof on the inside. The fact that the horse is inclined to brush should be mentioned to the blacksmith, who will then take care that the shoe is fitted close on the inside, or preferably use a three-quarter shoe.

Brushing boots, though not a remedy, may be necessary to protect the horse from injury.

Abscesses may be acute or chronic, caused by—

(1) Infection by bacteria.

(2) Thorns, splinters, pieces of metal, etc., embedded in the flesh.

(3) Disease, e.g., tuberculosis or fungoid growth.

Symptoms. Acute Abscesses. This is due to causes (1) or (2), and swelling, heat and tenderness are the conspicuous symptoms.

Treatment consists of encouraging the abscess to come to a head, which is accomplished by hot fomentations or by the use of Antiphlogistine.

If an abscess, after coming to a head, should prove stubborn and not burst, then veterinary aid should be called in as the use of the lance may be necessary.

After the abscess has burst, the cavity must be well syringed out with dilute disinfectant and treated as a deep wound.

Chronic Abscesses due to foreign bodies becoming capsuled or to disease feel cold and hard to the touch and are only slightly painful; they will not respond to fomentations and should be shown to the veterinary surgeon, as treatment varies according to the cause.

Poll Evil. The predisposing cause is a blow on the top of the head or continued pressure from a head collar.

Symptoms. A soft, painful swelling between the ears.

Treatment. This is the same as for an acute abscess, but owing to the position of the injury it is difficult to secure drainage.

Veterinary aid should be called in, as surgical treat-

H.H.O.   F

ment is the only possible method of dealing with the trouble.

Fistulous Wither. This is an abscess above the vertebræ at the wither which extends down between the shoulder blades. It is caused by a blow, a bite from another horse, or an ill-fitting collar or saddle. The

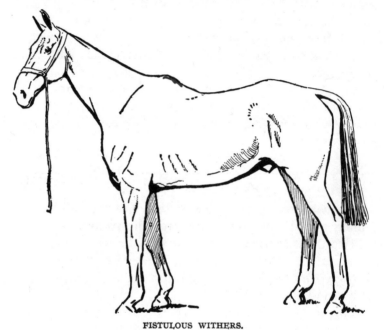

FISTULOUS WITHERS.

modern school of thought consider it is due to the abortion bacillus.

Symptoms. The first symptom is pain over the withers, followed by a swelling which may assume a large dimension. In most cases the swelling bursts, but in a few cases it will subside. If the swelling bursts, the skin may heal after the discharge has ceased, but this will be only temporary, and the abscess is sure to recur. Owing to the position of the abscess, it is extremely difficult to secure drainage, and the ligaments above the vertebræ are apt to be affected by the poison from the pus in the abscess.

Treatment. Fistulous withers is a very serious condition, and the veterinary surgeon should be called in immediately. He may be able to remove all diseased tissue by operation.

Neglected cases are often impossible to cure. The external application of poultices or blisters is useless.

Wounds of the Mouth. These are injuries caused by the bit. The bars of the mouth and the corners of the lips may be bruised or lacerated.

If the bars be badly injured it is quite likely that the nerves may remain permanently affected after the wound has healed, and this will give the horse a hard mouth.

If only one bar has been injured it will cause a one-sided mouth.

Bruises and wounds of this type are a frequent cause of a horse being shy about the head and not going kindly.

Treatment. Keep the bit out of the horse's mouth and bathe with a very dilute disinfectant—e.g., salt and water, or a bucket of water with $\frac{1}{2}$ teaspoonful of potassium permanganate added to it.

Burns and Scalds. The best treatment is to apply a solution of tannic acid or picric acid and bandage to exclude air.

These acids form a temporary skin and therefore relieve the pain. Another satisfactory treatment consists of Carron Oil.

Bleeding from the Nose. Due to a broken blood vessel and varies in degree. It will stop of its own accord as a rule, but is very likely to recur.

Treatment. Bathe the outside of the face over the nostrils with cold water or put on cold swabs. If the bleeding is from one nostril only this may be plugged with cotton wool. Calcium lactate given in the food may be used as a preventative.

Bleeding after Castration. This may occur after the veterinary surgeon has left.

Treatment. Get hold of the veterinary surgeon as soon as possible. Until he arrives cold water should be applied over the loins. This is conveniently done by placing a sack over the loins and keeping it wet with cold water.

If possible the wound should be plugged with cotton-wool which has been boiled in a saline solution or soaked in a dilute disinfectant.

Forging and Clicking. This noise is caused by the horse striking the toe of the fore foot with the toe of the hind foot.

It most frequently occurs when a horse is going slackly or is weak and unfit.

The only remedy is to keep the horse well collected and to have the shoes attended to.

The hind shoes should have the toe kept well back and the shoe of the fore foot should be rounded off.

CHAPTER IV

SKIN DISEASES

In this chapter it is intended to take the contagious diseases first as being the more important.

CONTAGIOUS

Mange. Parasitic mange is a disease scheduled under the Diseases of Animals Acts, and any suspicion of its existence must be reported to the local authorities immediately.

There are three forms :—

(1) Sarcoptic.

(2) Soroptic.

(3) Symbiotic.

The sarcoptic form is far the most serious. If once it gets a hold it is extremely difficult to eradicate and it does not yield readily to treatment.

An outbreak is particularly serious owing to its very infectious and contagious character. In a well-regulated private stable mange is not likely to occur. In the case of army horses on service an outbreak is serious owing to the alarming rapidity with which the disease spreads.

An infected horse must not be worked with or near others.

Sarcoptic mange may occur on any part of the body, but is usually found on the neck and withers.

Soroptic mange begins in the same way as sarcoptic, but is due to a different mite, which is distinguishable under the microscope and yields more readily to treatment.

Symbiotic mange is usually confined to the legs or root of the tail.

Symptoms. Intense irritation of the skin. The horse will evince signs of pleasure when scratched on the neck and shoulders with a stick. The affected parts become thickened and wrinkled, the hair eventually falling off, leaving the skin covered with small crusts.

Treatment. The treatment is the same for all kinds

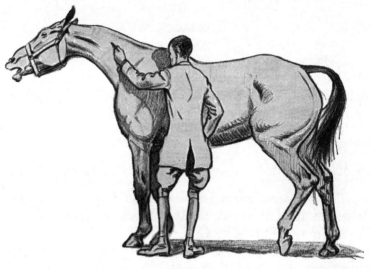

MANGE.

of mange. This must be energetic and disinfection of all in contact material rigidly enforced.

Isolate the horse at once and call in the veterinary surgeon. Put the horse on a cooling diet and clip him if necessary, burning every hair immediately. The bedding should also be burnt.

Great progress has been made lately in the treatment of mange by the use of D.D.T. preparations about which advice can be obtained from a veterinary surgeon.

Even if the animal appears to be cured, close observation must be kept as a recurrence is not unlikely.

All gear that is not wanted should be burnt, the remainder rigorously disinfected. The boxes occupied by the horse, both before and during treatment, should be washed from top to bottom with a strong disinfectant solution.*

Itchy Tail or Mane. These are irritations which may be due to a parasite or to a disordered condition of the blood. It is also often a symptom of worms.

In either case the horse will rub his tail or mane, causing the hair to drop out.

Treatment. If the complaint is due to a disordered condition of the blood, the affected parts should be washed with a mild solution of disinfectant * and a laxative * given, followed by a course of tonics.

The application of coconut oil will assist a cure.

If due to a parasite, the complaint should be treated in the same way as mange.

Ringworm is a highly contagious disease of the skin caused by a fungus.

Cause. Contagion. New horses, strange stables, railway boxes, etc., are all suspect, and, also, pre-infected clothing and saddlery.

Symptoms. The first symptoms are raised circular patches of hair, usually on the neck and shoulders; later the skin is left bare, leaving greyish white crusts.

It spreads very rapidly and will cause loss of condition.

Treatment. The horse must be isolated, and all gear and tackle thoroughly disinfected, that which is not of value being burnt.

If the coat is at all long the horse should be clipped (the hair being burnt at once). The actual ringworm patches should be washed with a warm solution of washing soda applied with a stiff nailbrush. After being allowed to dry apply *one* of the following *to the actual patches only* :—

* See Appendix, pages 134, 141.

        (a) Tr. Iodine
        (b) Blue Mercury Ointment
        (c) Iodoform Ointment

These dressings must be worked well into the patches, thoroughness being essential, since one incompletely treated patch will re-spread the infection.

The horse should be kept isolated and under observation for some time, for fear of a further outbreak.

Canadian Pox is a skin eruption consisting of clusters of pimples which may occur on any part of the body, but most frequently occur near the girths behind the elbow. It is a highly contagious disease and is due to a bacillus. The scabs come off, leaving bare patches of skin.

Treatment. Saturate cotton-wool with a solution of 1 part carbolic acid to 40 parts of water and dab on to the affected parts. A laxative diet is recommended.

Acne is a skin eruption rather similar to Canadian pox which occurs near the withers. It is highly contagious. The pimples are scattered and do not occur in clusters as in Canadian pox.

Treatment. Same as for Canadian pox.

Lice. These are found in horses in poor condition or in animals which have picked them up when out at grass.

They give rise to a blotchy appearance of the coat, and as they are blood-sucking animals they soon pull the horse back in condition.

Symptoms. The horse is seen to rub against any convenient object and on examination lice and nits will be seen. In the warmth of the sun lice can easily be seen on the surface of the coat.

Treatment. If possible clip out and groom thoroughly. Apply a Derris Root or D.D.T. preparation such as Pulvex and repeat in ten days so as to catch the eggs which have hatched out since the first application. Disinfectants are useless against lice and only blister the skin.

NON-CONTAGIOUS DISEASES

Humour. A pimply condition of the skin.
It is caused by a heated condition of the blood.
Symptoms. Pimples or pustules appear on any part of the body.
Treatment consists in seeing that the bowels are kept well open, and that the corn ration is not excessive.

Nettlerash. This complaint, also known as urticaria, consists of small areas of the skin becoming raised.
It is caused by errors of diet, stings or insect bites, and is non-contagious.
It occurs mostly in young animals or in horses kept idle in the stable and still getting their ordinary working diet.
The patches appear suddenly, and vary in size from a pea to a five-shilling piece.
The distribution is irregular and may extend over the whole body.
Treatment. The treatment is a purgative, bran mashes and a reduction of heating food.

Eczema. Eczema is an inflammation of the superficial layers of the skin; it is characterised by very small pimples, which may run together and emit a discharge.
It is often limited to a small area of the body.
It is non-contagious.
Its cause is not well known, but is believed to be due to dirt getting into the skin, chemical irritants or to indigestion.
Symptoms. Irritation may or may not be present. It takes one of two forms:—
(1) Dry eczema, in which the skin appears dry when the scale is picked off.
(2) Moist eczema, in which a liquid exudes from the small pimples causing a matting of the hair. This form generally causes irritation.

Eczema in the heels of a horse, or in the bend of the knee or hock, often assumes a scaly character, which is followed by the formation of ulcers. These are very painful and often cause severe lameness.

Treatment. Internal. Stop all heating food and substitute bran mashes with Epsom salts.

External. Clean the affected part and apply zinc ointment.

Cracked Heels and Mud Fever. These correspond to chapped hands in human beings and are inflammations of the skin on the heels, legs and possibly the belly. Cracked heels is really eczema of the heels.

Cause. They are both due to mud and wet, and a strong predisposing cause is washing a horse's legs after work.

Washing the legs and heels removes the natural oil and leaves the skin dry and brittle.

If the legs be bandaged loosely after hunting with flannel bandages and left to dry, then brushed out and rebandaged with clean flannel bandages, the trouble will not occur.

Mud fever is more prevalent in some districts than in others.

Horses with legs left unclipped are less prone to these complaints.

Treatment. Wash the legs well with warm soft water and white soap. Rinse and dry them *thoroughly*. Then apply the following lotion twice daily, dabbing it on with cotton-wool:—

Lead acetate	-	-	-	2 tablespoons.
Zinc sulphate	-	-	-	2 ,,
Glycerine	-	-	-	4 ,,
Water	-	-	-	1 quart.

The horse should be put on soft food, given a laxative and rested.

An alternative prescription is:—

Goulard's extract of lead -   2 tablespoons.
Olive oil -   -   -   -   1 pint.

Mix and apply daily.

As a preventive a little vaseline should be rubbed into the legs and heels before hunting.

Grease. This is more common in heavy horses, but may occur in light horses if cracked heels are not attended to.

It is frequently found in dirty stables, but should not occur in a well-managed establishment.

Symptoms. Cracks in the heel which become filled up with a cheesy-looking material.

There is a thin, foul and evil-smelling discharge.

In chronic cases grapes are formed on the skin.

Preventive Treatment. Do not wash the legs.

Treatment. The legs should be clipped and damped daily with a 1 per cent solution of zinc chloride.

They should also be kept bandaged with cotton wadding bandages in order to keep them warm and thus assist circulation.

A greasy heel, if firmly established, is very persistent and difficult to eradicate.

Heel Bug. As a rule only well-bred horses with thin skins are affected. The heels will be swollen and painful: lameness may also be present.

Treatment. Sulphanilamide ointment.

Warts are excrescences of the skin and occur most frequently on the nose, the inside of the hind leg and the sheath.

They are unsightly, though no detriment to the horse, unless in a position where the tackle rubs them.

Treatment. (1) A silk thread drawn tightly, and kept tight daily, round the base of a wart will generally cause it to drop off by arresting the flow of blood.

(2) A stick of caustic potash carefully applied may dissolve a wart, but generally veterinary aid is required.

Warbles. These are hard lumps which occur in the spring and early summer. They are not infectious as they are due to the maggot of the warble fly, which has laid its egg during the previous summer.

If the warble is situated under the saddle it is likely to cause trouble before the end of the hunting season, as its maturity is hastened by the warmth of the saddle.

Treatment. As soon as a warble is discovered the saddle must be kept off and fomentations applied to encourage the maggot to ripen.

When ripe a small hole can be felt in the centre of the lump through which the maggot will emerge, and this can be expedited by squeezing the base of the warble with both thumbs.

Undue pressure should not be exercised by the thumbs, or there is a danger of bursting the maggot under the skin.

Antiphlogistine will assist in bringing the warble to a head quickly.

After the warble has been evicted, the cavity should be washed with dilute disinfectant * and dressed with iodine.

Warbles not under the saddle or harness are not serious and will ripen naturally, but if a warble be burst under the skin, pressure, e.g., a saddle, will bring up a swelling until the dead tissue has been removed. This must be done by a veterinary surgeon.

Leucoderma is a name given to white patches which sometimes appear on the hairless parts of the horse, such as the parts round the eye and under the tail. They are due to lack of pigment, and apart from being unsightly are of no detriment.

Hidebound. This is not a disease but an indication

* See Appendix, page 134.

that the horse is suffering from worms or other internal disorder.

The skin appears dry and dull, and is inelastic to the touch.

Treatment. Treatment consists in getting rid of the cause. For a start give 1½ pints of linseed oil, and if no improvement is noticed, then have the horse treated for worms.

CHAPTER V

INTERNAL DISEASES

Cold in the Head. This is similar to a cold in human beings, and is brought about by exposure or infection. A cold in itself is not a serious complaint, but it is most important that it should be noticed in its early stages and that the horse should be rested. Serious complications such as pneumonia frequently follow when a horse has been worked with a cold.

Symptoms. Sneezing is often one of the first symptoms and the horse appears to be dull and lethargic.

There is a thin discharge from the nose which, after a short time, becomes thick. The horse will probably have a cough.

The eyes may water and the coat will be dull and staring.

The horse may be slightly feverish, but if the temperature does not subside in a few days it is a sign of complications.

Treatment. The horse should be put on a laxative diet and as much nitre as will go on a sixpence added to his water once a day.

The stable should be well ventilated, but free from draughts and the horse warmly rugged up.

Inhalations of eucalyptus * should be given to assist the discharge from the nostrils. Make free use of the thermometer and on no account work the horse if it has any temperature.

Coughs. One of the most troublesome complaints that can start in a stable is coughing, and many horses are laid up for a considerable time owing to it. A cough

* See Appendix, page 140.

is not in itself a disease, but one of the symptoms of several troubles.

As treatment varies with the cause, it is essential to diagnose correctly the cause of the cough. Coughing is very likely to start in a stable when horses have been brought in from grass, and in this case it is due to the impure air of the stable or indigestion. The prevention of a cough of this kind lies in keeping the stable door open night and day, and in making the change from soft to hard food gradual and not sudden.

Horses very seldom cough when turned out to grass even if the weather is wet and cold.

Any form of cough is an unsoundness in a horse as long as it persists.

In cases of throat or lung trouble medicines must never be administered in the form of a drench. They should be given in the food, water or in the form of an electuary.

Sore Throat Cough. See Laryngitis.

Cough due to Irritants. Another cause of cough is that due to a drench, some of which has gone down the windpipe instead of the gullet, or to an irritant, such as a thistle, which has stuck in the throat.

Coughs due to these causes will probably right themselves in a short time, but if a considerable quantity of fluid has got into the lungs the irritation may give rise to pneumonia and must be treated as such.

Cough due to Indigestion. Coughs due to indigestion are frequently described as long and drawn out. They are due to discomfort in the stomach and intestines, and are frequently accompanied by an unthrifty appearance and a dull, staring coat.

Treatment. This consists in removal of the cause. It is as well to see the effect of $1\frac{1}{2}$ pints of linseed oil. In many cases this will do the trick, but if no improvement is noticed, worms should be suspected as the cause of the trouble and the horse fasted and dosed for worms.

Cough due to Broken Wind. This form is chronic and is another long-drawn-out cough. The only form of treatment is palliative, which consists in giving all the food damp, and following out the instructions given for broken wind.

Cough due to Teething. Teething may upset the general health of a young horse and cause a cough.

This cough will disappear as soon as the cause has disappeared, and the only treatment necessary is to keep the bowels well open by the addition of Epsom salts * to the food.

Laryngitis, which is similar to sore throat in man, may assume a serious phase in a horse. It is an inflammation of the inner lining of the throat which will cause a cough, a discharge from the nostrils and difficulty in breathing.

Externally the throat will be swollen and a harsh sound will be noticeable as the horse breathes. In very severe cases the horse may choke owing to the air passage being blocked, in which case death follows.

Treatment. The horse must be kept warm with plenty of clothing and the stable well ventilated.

Eucalyptus inhalations * should be given, and camphor and belladonna electuary * smeared on the tongue three or four times daily.

The throat should be rubbed with liniment.

The horse probably will not take its food, owing to the soreness in the throat, so he should be encouraged to take nourishment in the form of gruel or linseed tea.

As soon as he will eat, bran mashes should be given, and he is more likely to nibble grass than hay. If green food is not available, the hay should be damped.

Bronchitis. This is an inflammation of the throat and bronchial tubes.

* See Appendix, pages 141, 140, 142.

It is caused by—

(1) Bacteria.

(2) Chemical or mechanical irritants.

(3) Exposure to cold, especially when the animal is in an exhausted condition.

Symptoms. A harsh dry cough, which is increased by exercise. As the disease progresses the cough will become softer. A discharge from the nostrils, thin and watery at the outset, later becomes thick.

The temperature may rise to 105° F.

The pulse is fast and soft.

The respiration is quick and laboured.

There is a discharge from the eyes, and the mucous membranes are dull red in colour.

Treatment. On no account should physic balls or drenches be given, as these are apt to choke the animal or set up pneumonia. Plenty of air is essential, warmth being provided by rugs and bandages.

Inhalations of eucalyptus * will give relief.

Hot fomentations * should be applied to the chest wall.

The throat should be rubbed with liniment.

It is advisable to call in the veterinary surgeon.

Asthma. This disease is very rare in the horse. When it occurs the condition is chronic and the breathing becomes distressed at more or less regular intervals.

The cause is not certain, but may be due to insanitary or stuffy stables.

Treatment. There is no satisfactory treatment, but it is advisable to give all food damp, as in the case of broken wind.

Strangles. An acutely contagious disease of the nose and throat. In severe cases there is always swelling and suppuration of the submaxillary glands, while in extreme cases the same may occur in other parts of the body.

H.H.O.   * See Appendix, pages 140, 139.   G

The disease is caused by an organism called the streptococcus of strangles. It most frequently attacks young horses. The chief cause of an attack is infection by means of forage, infected mangers or stables, railway boxes, or by paddocks infected with the disease.

Infected bedding, head collars, buckets, grooming kit, etc., may also be the cause of this disease, which spreads with lightning rapidity. Fresh air, suitable food

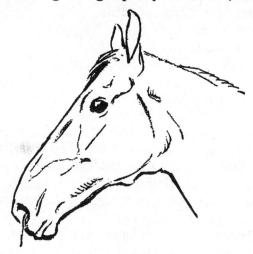

STRANGLES

and adequate exercise, combined with strict and hygienic stable management, will do much to prevent its occurrence.

Symptoms. The first noticeable signs will be dullness and apathy, together with a rise of temperature, probably to between 103° and 105° F. The mucous membrane of the eye will be found on examination to be an unhealthy red colour, as opposed to the light pink of the healthy horse.

A thin watery discharge from one or both nostrils will turn to a thick, yellowish one. There may be sore throat and coughing. The glands beneath the throat will swell and become very hot and tender. Later they will soften and burst, whereupon the temperature will quickly fall.

The danger is that, should the organism penetrate to and infect the blood stream (Bastard strangles), abscesses may be formed in the lungs, liver, spleen, kidneys or brain, in which case death will follow. Abscesses may also form on joints or tendons. These of themselves are not fatal, though they may lead to chronic lameness.

In this case the swelling of the submaxillary glands is less pronounced.

Strangles occurs most frequently in horses under six years old.

Treatment. Because of the highly contagious nature of the disease treatment must concern not only the patient but all other horses in the stables or vicinity. To this end the patient should be isolated in a roomy, airy box, well ventilated and free from draughts. The old box must be most carefully disinfected, as must every article of clothing, saddlery and equipment which has or may have been in contact with the sick horse.

Keep the patient warm by means of rugs and flannel bandages—not by shutting doors and windows.

Give inhalations of eucalyptus.*

Cleanse the nostrils frequently with warm water and keep them smeared with eucalyptus ointment. The membranes of the nostrils are extremely sensitive, and even a weak solution of disinfectant will aggravate the trouble.

Abscesses should be encouraged to mature by the application of some stimulating liniment. If their bursting is delayed the veterinary surgeon should be summoned, since, should they burst internally, the blood stream may be affected, with dire results. When the

* See Appendix, page 140.

abscesses do burst they should be treated as ordinary wounds.

Food should be soft and easily digested. Green food, steamed hay, a very little crushed oats, linseed mash, carrots or turnips may be varied and given in such a way as will tempt the horse to eat.

The disease runs its course in from four to six weeks and the period of convalescence is a long one—two months at least. A further long period of conditioning will be necessary before normal work can be resumed.

Wind trouble is a not infrequent sequel to strangles.

Vaccine treatment is necessary for Bastard strangles.

Congestion of the Lungs. This is due to the presence of an abnormal quantity of blood in the lungs. As it is frequently followed by pneumonia unless attended to, it is most advisable to seek expert assistance at once.

There are a number of causes which bring on congestion of the lungs:—

(1) The presence of bacteria.

(2) Chemical irritants, e.g., medicines.

(3) Exposure to bad weather.

(4) Cardiac debility. This frequently follows hard exercise if a horse is unfit, and is not uncommon at the end of a long hunt or if a horse is ridden to a standstill.

Symptoms. If it occurs in the hunting field the symptoms are alarming.

The horse is likely to fall if pressed to move. Respiration is very exaggerated, and the flanks and chest wall will heave.

The horse will stand with legs outstretched and the head and neck extended.

The nostrils are dilated and the animal is in a staggering condition. The mucous membrane of the eye is a dull bluish colour and the pulse weak. The temperature will probably rise rapidly as high as 106° F. and the animal may break out into a cold sweat.

First-aid Treatment. If in the hunting field turn the sick animal with his head to the wind, remove girths, throat lash, etc., and throw a coat over his back. Stand him still and do not move him for at least half an hour. The old-fashioned remedy of giving whisky or brandy diluted is out-dated.

Treatment. Place the horse in an airy box, clothe warmly and feed with laxative and nutritious food, which must not be of a bulky nature and send for the veterinary surgeon.

A long period of convalescence is necessary.

Pneumonia. This is inflammation of the lungs and is due to the same causes as congestion. It frequently follows influenza or strangles, or may be caused by senility, anæmia or debility.

Symptoms. Breathing is difficult and hurried, the head is outstretched and the nostrils dilated. The temperature will be above normal and the mucous membrane of the eye have a bluish colour.

The pulse is rapid and weak.

There may be a cough and a thin nasal discharge.

The patient may have shivering attacks.

A horse seldom lies down during an attack of acute pneumonia.

If the disease progresses favourably the temperature will gradually subside, but a sudden drop of the temperature is a very bad sign.

In advanced stages the colour of the nasal discharge becomes yellowish brown.

The animal is generally constipated and the fæces may be mucus-coated.

Treatment. As in all pulmonary diseases, nursing is of the greatest importance. The patient should be well rugged up and bandaged, and plenty of fresh air allowed to enter the box.

Eucalyptus inhalations * may be given, and the bowels kept open with 4 tablespoonfuls of Epsom salts in the drinking water daily.

As much nitre as will go on a sixpence may also be given daily in the drinking water.

The horse *should not be drenched.*

It is a most serious illness and veterinary aid should be called in as early as possible.

Pleurisy. This is an inflammation of the pleura or membrane covering the lungs.

It is usually caused by bacterial infection, but may also follow a wound in the wall of the chest.

Symptoms. The horse is off its feed.

The patient appears to be distressed and in pain, and is unwilling to move as movement increases the pain. The pulse is hard and fast.

The temperature will be high, up to 107° F.

There may be a discharge from the eyes and nose.

The breathing is fast, and the flank and abdomen work excessively, while the chest does not appear to move.

The patient seldom lies down.

The course of the disease is rapid, and death may follow in two or three days. In some cases, however, it is more protracted. Pneumonia is a usual complication.

Treatment. As in pneumonia, keep the patient in an airy box and maintain warmth with plenty of clothing and bandages.

Hot poultices or a mild blister * may be applied to the chest wall.

Epsom salts (4 tablespoonfuls) and nitre (1 teaspoonful) should be given in the drinking water daily.

The veterinary surgeon should be sent for. It may be necessary to tap the chest to withdraw fluid.

Contagious Pleuro-pneumonia. This disease is for-

* See Appendix, pages 140, 139.

tunately not very common, but serious outbreaks occur from time to time. It is due to bacterial infection gaining access to the lungs during inhalation or through food and water which has been in contact with an infected animal.

It has a period of incubation of two to seven days.

Symptoms. At first the animal does not go off its feed, but appears listless and may have a cough.

The temperature will rise as high as 106° F.

The appetite disappears and the respirations become rapid and laboured.

The mucous membrane of the eye becomes vivid red.

There is a discharge from the nostrils, thin and watery at first, which later becomes thick and brown in colour.

The patient will grunt. A swelling is present under the chest.

The crisis is reached about the sixth day.

As a horse is unlikely to recover if it has been worked in the earliest stages immediate diagnosis is essential to successful treatment.

Treatment. Rigid isolation.

Relief may be given by eucalyptus inhalations.*

The best foods to give are steamed hay, boiled oats, linseed mash, gruel or fresh grass.

A long period of convalescence is required.

The veterinary surgeon should be called in.

Influenza. The influenzas of man and other animals are entirely different diseases from the influenza of the horse.

The actual origin of the disease is unknown, but it is highly infectious and is spread by contagion, clothing, food, bedding, grooming kit or infected stables.

To avoid the spread of this disease everything which

* See Appendix, page 140.

may have been in contact must be thoroughly disinfected.

Influenza has a period of incubation of two to five days, and after the symptoms become apparent may turn into either—

(1) *The mild type*, which will run its course in six to eight days, or

(2) *The severe type or pinkeye*, in which the most critical period is the fifth to the eighth day.

Symptoms. In both types the patient has a high temperature and is in an exhausted condition.

There will be a catarrhal discharge from eyes and nostrils, great depression, coughing and a high temperature, which should gradually decline.

If the temperature, which is normally high at the commencement, does not gradually subside the outlook is not very hopeful.

The severe type or pinkeye is recognised by the bright red colour of the eye as opposed to the dirty yellowish colour produced by the mild type, and is often complicated by pneumonia.

The legs, muzzle and belly may be swollen.

Apart from fatal results, which are common with this disease, the great danger lies in the very possible legacy of permanent respiratory trouble.

Treatment. Prevention is far better than cure, and a really healthy horse is far less liable to the disease than one run down and in poor condition.

If an outbreak of influenza occurs in the stable, the temperature of every horse should be taken daily before work, as in mild cases a rise of temperature is the earliest symptom.

Good stable management, isolation of new horses, care when travelling and subsequent isolation will assist in keeping the disease away.

If, in spite of precautions, influenza occurs, isolate the

patient at once in a roomy, airy box free from draughts, rug up well and bandage the legs.

Really careful nursing is of the greatest importance.

Give soft food little and often.

Steam the head frequently with inhalations of eucalyptus.*

As pneumonia is a frequent sequel to even the mild form of influenza it is advisable to call in your veterinary surgeon.

Constipation. Put on soft food, give a laxative and an enema if necessary.

It is due to faulty feeding and lack of exercise, and its recurrence should be avoided by giving laxative food and small doses of salts.

Diarrhœa Purging and Superpurgation. Diarrhœa is not necessarily a symptom of disease, as it may be an effort to dislodge or expel indigestible or injurious matter. It is due to a variety of causes, e.g.:

(1) Sudden changes of diet (such as turning out to grass without preparation).

(2) The presence of red worms in the intestine.

(3) Chill on the stomach.

(4) Excitement.

Purging as a result of physic is not a disease.

Superpurgation is the result of an overdose of physic or of the physic having been administered without suitable preparation.*

Treatment. Diarrhœa must be treated in a way that will remove the cause. If it is due to injurious matter in the stomach or intestine the first thing to do is to give a pint of linseed oil. This will assist to lubricate the intestines and pass out the irritant matter. Once the irritant has been removed 1 to 4 drachms of chlorodyne and ½ oz. of bismuth may be given in flour gruel.

* See Appendix, pages 140, 141.

Superpurgation. Give 1 to 4 drachms of chlorodyne and ½ oz. of bismuth.

A frequent sequel of superpurgation is constipation; therefore, as soon as the purging has ceased, small doses of salts should be given in mashes.

Colic. This familiar disease is similar to stomach ache in man and the pain varies in intensity.

The condition is caused by—

(1) Over-taxing the stomach with food.

(2) A stoppage in the S bend between the stomach and the small intestine.

(3) Parasites.

(4) Digestive troubles.

(5) Easily fermented foods, e.g., new oats, mouldy hay, etc.

(6) Indiscreet watering.

(7) Twisted gut.

(8) Sand in the stomach.

(9) Stones in the bowels, kidneys or bladder.

Symptoms. The horse appears uneasy in the stable, off his food, looks round at his flank and may break into a profuse sweat. Respiration is laboured; the pulse is quick and accentuated; the mucous membrane of the eye is much inflamed; there may be straining to pass fæces and urine.

The horse will look round and kick at his stomach.

He will repeatedly lie down and get up again. When down he may roll with considerable violence. The temperature may rise a degree or two, but the surest indication is the pulse.

Twisted gut is a form of colic which is caused by a stumble, a fall or by too heavy a feed in the case of an animal brought home after a long day's work.

The opinion is often expressed that the horse by rolling causes a twist. It is at least as likely that a twist causes rolling. In the case of a twist the temperature may rise to 105°, which is higher than in other forms of colic.

Treatment. If on the road the horse wants to stop and appears uneasy, colic will probably be the cause, and the first thing to be done by the rider is to get the horse into a box and encourage staling. Shake straw up under the belly and whistle.

On arrival home, put the horse in a large and airy box and bed well down.

Administer a colic drink or the following:—

Turpentine - - - -	2 tablespoonfuls.
Linseed oil - - - -	1½ pints.
Whisky or brandy - -	2 tablespoonfuls.

The horse may roll, but must be watched to avoid injury.

A hot blanket rolled up and applied under the belly well back will help to reduce pain and stimulate the action of the bowels, as will a warm enema.

If the patient is not better in an hour after the drench is administered the veterinary surgeon should be sent for.

It is advisable to keep a stock of colic drinks which have been made up by your veterinary surgeon.

Worms. Horses are particularly susceptible to attack by various forms of these parasites, which are known collectively as worms.

A. Stomach Bots. These are not true worms but arise from the attack of a yellowish-brown fly—the gad-fly or bot-fly—which lays its eggs on the legs when the horse is out at grass. The legs are then licked by the animal and the eggs are thus transferred to the stomach, where they hatch out into the larvæ known as stomach bots.

Symptoms. Few horses are entirely free from bots, and they are not injurious except in very large quantities, when they cause loss of condition and even debility, together with a staring and dry coat. A horse which, eating a good ration, does not thrive, may be suspected of bots.

Bots, which are about $\frac{3}{4}$ inch in length, may be expelled with the dung.

Treatment. If large quantities of eggs are seen the legs may be clipped and the hair burnt—or the legs may be singed with a singeing lamp. An animal affected internally by the parasite should be starved for twenty-four hours, when a drench consisting of 2 tablespoonfuls of turpentine in 1 pint of linseed oil should be given.

B. Common Intestinal or Round Worm. This is the commonest of all worms, being found in most domestic animals. That found in the horse is white, stiff and up to a foot in length, and is generally about as thick as a pencil.

Symptoms. In small numbers these rarely give rise to any symptoms, but in large numbers they may cause stoppage or irregularity of the bowels, loss of condition and intermittent colic.

Treatment. Starve the horse for at least twenty-four hours—even thirty-six hours is not too much in an aggravated case—then drench with 2 to 4 tablespoonfuls of turpentine to 1 pint of linseed oil. If this has no effect call in the veterinary surgeon, who will give an intestinal lavage (stomach pump) with saline solution or other preparation.

If the horse is at grass a change of pasture is advisable after treatment.

C. Red Worm. The red worm is a blood-sucker, and is therefore by far the most harmful of all parasites which attack the horse. Moreover, they pass through the bowel wall into the blood vessels, causing stoppage of the blood stream. This results eventually in symptoms of colic or a blood-clot.

They are reddish in colour and up to $\frac{1}{2}$ inch long.

Symptoms. These are most alarming, especially in young horses, and include loss of flesh, anæmia, hollow flanks, dropped abdomen and dry coat.

The action of the bowels is irregular, and in most cases a particularly offensive diarrhœa is present. The mucous membrane of the eye is very pale and the appetite is variable. The worm may be visible if the droppings are carefully examined but such is not always the case and the degree of infection can only be ascertained with accuracy by a microscopic count of the number of worm eggs in a given area. If not treated excessive debility will set in and the horse will eventually be unable to rise.

Treatment. If the animal is at grass he should be taken up and given highly nutritious diet. Phenothiozine powder is the latest method of treatment and control; this has superceded all former drugs as the safest and most effective. It is given either as a powder in the feed (without fasting) or dissolved in water as a drench, but better still by the stomach tube, as by this method the exact amount given can be assured. The dose varies from 10 grammes in a foal to 30 grammes for a full-grown horse in fair condition. Care should be taken not to exceed these doses as some horses appear to be more susceptible than others to the drug and bad results may occur. The dose should also not be repeated under three weeks. A microscopic "worm count" should be taken after treatment to ensure that it has been successful.

D. Whip Worms are about $1\frac{3}{4}$ inches in length and very thin. They occur in the rectum.

Symptoms. The horse will rub his tail and a sticky discharge will be visible at the anus.

Treatment. A handful of salt in a gallon of warm water should be given as an enema.

Congestion of the Kidneys. Congestion of the kidneys is due to the failure of the kidneys to excrete impure substances which enter the blood during the course of fevers such as glanders, to tuberculosis or to feeding mouldy hay, fermented grain or the like.

The condition may also arise as the result of shock or injuries in the neighbourhood of the loins, or as the result of chill.

Symptoms. There is an increase in the amount of urine passed, which will also be of a lighter colour than normal. There is also stiffness of movement, especially in the hind quarters, and the horse will show tenderness to pressure over the loins.

Treatment. (1) Keep the patient warmly rugged and bandaged, and at rest.

(2) A change of diet may be indicated; the food should consist chiefly of linseed mashes.

(3) If the condition can be traced to defective foodstuffs an aloetic ball should be given. If due to other causes an aperient should not be given.

Stones in the Kidneys. These seldom give rise to much trouble unless both kidneys are affected.

Symptoms. Colicky pains after work. Tenderness to pressure over the loins. Repeated attempts to stale. Sandy or gritty deposits in urine.

Treatment. Give plenty of fluids. Add a dessertspoonful of bicarbonate of soda to each bucket of drinking water.

Stones in the Bladder. Small stones may give rise to no symptoms; larger ones give rise to colicky pains and stiffness of gait. They are apt to increase in size with age, and frequently end by the sudden death of the animal.

The urine may dribble continually and be mixed with blood.

The urine is of a high colour and smells of ammonia.

Treatment. This can only be palliative. A warm enema may be given.

Veterinary advice should be sought, as an operation may be possible.

Stones in the Intestines. These are due to deposits of lime salts in the bowels, which may reach a great size. Medium-sized calculi about the size of a cricket ball are most dangerous as they may shift and cause a complete stoppage.

Symptoms. Repeated attacks of colic, which eventually prove fatal. There is no cure.

Azoturia (Monday Morning Disease). The true cause of this disease is not known.

It is due to enforced idleness of a horse in hard condition if the ration of corn is not reduced.

Symptoms. A rolling motion becomes apparent shortly after leaving the stable, there is stiffness in the hind quarters and the horse may drag his hind legs. There is excessive perspiration, and the muscles can be seen quivering. If the horse be forced to proceed he may fall down and be unable to rise. He may become violent.

The muscles of the loins may become very hard and tense, and the temperature rises two or three degrees to about 103° F. There will be quickened breathing. If any urine is passed, it will be coffee coloured. Mild cases quickly recover; severe cases are followed by death in a few days. Another sequel may be pneumonia of a fatal type.

Treatment. The malady can be prevented by suitable diet in the case of enforced rest.

When a horse is found to be suffering from azoturia he must be got home at once in a horse box and a warm enema given. He must not be walked more than is absolutely essential. Hot blankets should be applied to the loins and a veterinary surgeon sent for. The food during treatment should be of a laxative nature.

Lampas. This is a swollen condition of the roof of the mouth, and is generally associated with cutting of the permanent teeth.

The old treatment of slitting the roof of the mouth

or rubbing salt into the roof of the mouth is not recommended.

A laxative should be given and followed by a course of Epsom salts in the drinking water or food, to improve the condition of the blood.

Anthrax. is caused by a bacillus and is a notifiable disease. It is always fatal and generally runs a rapid course, the animal dying in a few hours.

Symptoms. (1) Very high temperature.

(2) Abnormal swellings of the throat and neck.

(3) Great pain.

There is no cure.

Shivering is a nervous affection characterised by involuntary and spasmodic muscular contractions.

The horse will generally cringe when touched along the back. Its hind limbs seem out of control and the horse backs with great difficulty.

A forelimb, lips, eyes or neck may be affected.

It is a slowly progressing disease and may follow serious illness or a bad fall.

It is incurable.

Megrims or Staggers. This is the name given to an affection of the brain resulting in sudden loss of equilibrium. It corresponds to fainting in the human being.

It is due to—

(*a*) Defective circulation caused by a weak heart, or by undue restraint of throat lash, collar, etc.

(*b*) Impaired digestion, the result of incorrect feeding.

(*c*) Congestion of the brain.

(*d*) Worms.

Symptoms. Attacks arise almost always while the horse is at work. They are periodical, at intervals of months or years.

The horse will halt, sway, stagger and finally fall to the ground unconscious.

Consciousness usually returns fairly quickly, when

the animal will get up and appear dazed. The attack lasts about five minutes.

Treatment. Remove all possible causes of restraint, such as bridles, collars, etc. Apply cold water to the head. As treatment varies with the cause, the veterinary surgeon should be called in. If expert advice is unobtainable and the attack is due to cause (*a*) an ammonia drench * should be given and no purgative; if due to (*b*), (*c*) or (*d*) an aloetic ball should be given, followed by treatment for worms if necessary.

Rheumatism. Acute rheumatism as known in man is extremely rare in the horse. If it occurs, the lameness is likely to shift from one limb to another, and may appear in the knee one day and the hock the next.

Treatment. Rheumatism is due to salts of uric acid in the blood, hence green food and a generally laxative diet is indicated.

If the lameness is not severe, gentle exercise may be given. In the stable the horse should be warmly rugged up and weak embrocation well massaged into the affected limb.

Arthritis. This disease, which is not uncommon, is unfortunately incurable, though it may be of long duration. It occurs mainly in old horses, and its cause is not known. In the early stages it may be extremely difficult to diagnose, as the horse may be sound one day and lame the next. Gradually the lameness will become more persistent until eventually the horse will be unworkable. As the disease eats away the bone, it makes a rough surface for the tendon or the opposing bone to work over.

Arthritis may occur anywhere from the shoulder or stifle to the foot.

Concussion of the Brain. Any blow of sufficient severity, such as knocking the head violently against a low beam in the stable, or against a low stable door, running into a tree, wall, etc., may cause concussion.

Symptoms. Loss of consciousness (which may or may not return after a short interval). The pupils are dilated; breathing is laboured and irregular; the action of the bowels and the bladder is involuntary.

Paralysis may occur after the patient recovers consciousness.

Treatment. Absolute quiet. Cold water should be poured over the head and spine. A stimulant such as ammonia placed to the nostrils may be administered. The veterinary surgeon should be sent for.

Joint Evil. This disease affects foals from birth till eighteen months old. If it develops within twenty-four hours of birth it is probably due to infection in the uterus before birth.

The disease is caused by bacterial infection through the navel, or through the mare's milk, and is due to a variety of organisms.

Symptoms. These vary according to the virulence of the organism causing the disease. The general symptoms are—

(1) An indisposition to suckle.

(2) A rise of temperature from normal 100° F. to about 103° F.

(3) Stiffness of movement and possible swelling of the joints, particularly those of the stifle, knee, hock and elbow.

(4) Signs of the infection at the navel—e.g., swelling, discharge or abscesses.

(5) Lameness, bowel irregularity, and a marked tendency to lie down. In many cases death follows, those foals which recover being backward for a long period.

Treatment. This is mainly preventive. The navel must be thoroughly disinfected at birth with iodine solution and the cord tied with a silk thread near the belly. If foaling takes place in a box, this should be most care-fully disinfected—preferably by blow-lamp—before the mare is put in to foal. The disease is less often found in the case of mares allowed to foal out of doors.

Where the disease is prevalent vaccine treatment of the in-foal mare should be tried.

This is a most serious complaint, and the veterinary surgeon should be sent for on the least suspicion of ailing on the part of the foal.

Biliary Fever. This fever is fortunately not found in England, but it is prevalent in many countries and was the cause of great mortality among the British army horses in Egypt and Salonika during the war.

Biliary fever is due to a microbe which gains entrance to the blood stream of the horse through a tick.

Symptoms. The horse which appeared well is suddenly noticed to have the symptoms of jaundice, the mucous membrane of the eye and nostrils is yellow, the heart weak and the temperature high—103° to 106°.

The animal appears very distressed and the hind legs may be swollen. Extreme debility is produced by this fever in a very short time.

In severe cases a sudden collapse after a few days is followed by death.

Treatment. In climates where ticks are prevalent a daily search should be made and all ticks removed from the horse.

In some cases a cure will be effected if the animal be kept warm and well nursed, every effort being made to encourage the patient to take nourishment while the fever is running its course. Injections of a preparation of quinine hydrobromide direct into the veins may be effective if the case is taken in hand early.

This must be done by a veterinary surgeon.

CHAPTER VI

WIND, HEART AND EYE

IT must be remembered that "whistling" and "roaring" are different degrees of the same complaint, namely, an affection of the larynx or throat due to paralysis of the left vocal cord.

Broken wind is a different disease affecting the lungs only.

The paralysis decreases the available area of inhalation, and the actual noise is caused by the forcible passage of air through a restricted aperture.

A horse starts the process of "going in the wind" by "whistling," and the odds are that later on—it may be soon or it may not be for some years—he will generally become a "roarer."

The horse is not getting enough air into its lungs and lack of staying power is usually the sequel. Distress from "roaring" may lead to heart trouble. "Whistling" generally commences in horses under six years of age, but older ones are not immune from it.

Testing a Horse for His Wind. Whistling may be heard at the trot, but the best way to test a horse for his wind is to have him trotted and cantered on a small circle, wearing his usual bridle.

This should be done on both reins, and as the horse comes close by you listen very carefully for any noise as he takes his breath.

Then have the horse galloped and pulled up near you and listen again. Some horses will make a noise at slow paces only, and more when going on one rein than on the other. There is a diversity of opinion as to whether the horse should be ridden by the examiner or not, but it is safest to do so, especially if nothing is heard when unmounted. The fitter the horse is, the less noise he will make.

Grunting. If, in the stable, you threaten to hit a horse in the flanks and he grunts, he must be regarded with suspicion, as often grunting and unsound wind go together, though not invariably.

Unless you have experience yourself it is wise to have him "grunted" by an expert, as there are some " grunts " which constitute unsoundness and others which do not, and there is a subtle difference between the two.

Thick in the Wind. A horse will often be thick in the wind when he is gross and fat, and in this condition should not be given severe or fast work, as it might lead to whistling. A gross horse may convey the impression of being wrong in the wind when not so in actual fact. Thick wind may be a sequel to bronchitis, or may be a temporary condition, but as long as it persists it is an unsoundness.

High Blowing. A noise made by horses during exhalation only. It is caused by a flapping of the nostrils and may lead the uninitiated into suspecting unsoundness in the wind. High blowers are usually very sound-winded horses. High blowing is due to an abnormality of the false nostril and is not a disease; in fact, it is quite common among well-bred horses.

Whistling. This is a high-pitched note generally heard in fast paces. It does not cause much harm in the case of a hunter, but is serious as it generally turns, sooner or later, into roaring.

Intermittent Whistlers. A horse is called an intermittent whistler when one day he makes a noise and another day he is sound, or he may vary from hour to hour. This undoubtedly is a weakness of nervous origin, and though the horse may pass the veterinary surgeon, it is more than probable that one day he will be a real "whistler."

Pronounced Roarers. These make a deep noise as they draw in their breath at any kind of fast work, and if really galloped become so distressed that they have to be pulled up.

Symptoms. Roaring may be heard when the horse is galloped, trotted or cantered. It may be scarcely perceptible or quite noticeable, according to the gravity of the condition.

Treatment of Whistling and Roaring. Once the condition has definitely been established it generally gets worse by degrees and no preventive treatment is of much use. A horse kept fit will make less noise than when unfit.

The best remedy is an operation and the earlier it is done the better the chance of its being successful.

The operation consists of stripping the lining membrane from the pouch which is behind the vocal chord and allowing the cords to adhere to the walls of the larynx so as to leave the air space permanently open.

This operation has been performed in England on thousands of horses in the last thirty years and in many cases has worked a complete and permanent cure.

Even if a complete cure does not result the horse which before operating was useless will probably become a workably sound animal.

Broken Wind is over-distention and a breakdown of the air vesicles of the lungs caused by too much strain being put on them. This may occur in a chronic cough or after bronchitis, asthma, pleurisy or pneumonia.

It may be brought about by excessive feeding before exercise, especially on bulky foods like sanfoin, vetches, lucerne or dusty hay, and it is for this reason that horses that make a habit of eating their bedding should be muzzled.

During even moderate exercise the horse appears distressed.

Symptoms. In the early stages the horse has a harsh, dry cough, which gets worse with exercise, and there is a slight discharge from the nose.

Later the cough becomes weak and short, and after any exertion the breathing is unduly laboured.

If the horse sneezes after a bout of coughing it is a good sign, as it means that the cough is probably only due to some irritation of the throat.

The effect of broken wind is to cause an alteration in the breathing, as instead of breathing in and out regularly, on exhalation there will be a sort of double effort to force out the breath. This can best be noticed by watching the flanks, when it will be observed that the horse appears to heave twice on exhalation. Broken wind is also called "Heaves" for this reason.

The condition and shape of a horse with broken wind changes; the animal will develop a large stomach, and the flanks will fall away.

Treatment. There is nothing that will cure a broken-winded horse, but in the early stages a great deal can be done to ease matters by special feeding. All food should be damp and linseed oil mixed with it two or three times a week. It is advisable to call in the veterinary surgeon to obtain advice as to the feeding and treatment of the particular case.

This disease is not considered hereditary.

THE HEART

In recent years, far more attention has been paid to heart conditions: in a veterinary surgeon's examination for soundness particular attention is now paid to the heart. Some of the symptoms which may point to heart diseases are: inability to stay, tiring easily when fit, loss of condition and irregular pulse. The owner of a horse that has developed any of these symptoms (which had not been noticed previously) should have the heart examined by a veterinary surgeon who will be able to advise whether to continue working the horse or not. Not all horses with irregular hearts are unsafe rides and many cases may continue in quite safe regular work for years whereas others are quite unsafe to ride. It should be remembered that a horse's heart may also be strained in the same way as that of an athlete that is by too much fast work before he is fit; in the same way many "roarers" have unsound hearts hence the advisability of an early operation in these cases. With an old horse it is a wise precaution to have its heart tested annually.

THE EYE

Sight is very important to the horse, as indeed it is to nearly every mammal, and as the more serious diseases are difficult for the amateur to detect the warranty of a hunter at auction guarantees soundness of the eye as well as wind.

Conjunctivitis and Opacity of the Cornea. The commonest diseases of the eye are—

(1) *Conjunctivitis*, which is an inflammation of the membrane covering the eye, called the conjunctiva.

(2) *Corneal Opacity.*

Either of these may be due to any of the following causes:—

(a) Cold.

(b) The presence of foreign matter in the eye.

(c) A blow or flick from a whip lash.

WIND, HEART AND EYE 117

Symptoms. Tears are visible and the affected eye is swollen. The eye will probably be kept closed to protect it from the light.

If it is due to cold both eyes may be affected.

The cornea, which in health is quite transparent, may show a speck or whip mark.

Later it may become dim, having a cloudy appearance like steamy glass.

Treatment. The eye must be carefully examined for the presence of any foreign body, which if present must be carefully removed. The eye may then be bathed with boracic lotion and the eyelid smeared with boracic ointment or vaseline.

The patient should be kept in a dark box on a laxative diet.

Epsom salts* may be given in the drinking water to keep the bowels open.

Ophthalmia. This is an inflammation of the eyeball and may be due to a blow or to infection.

It is an extremely painful condition and in only a few cases is recovery complete.

Frequently cataract or complete loss of sight follows this complaint.

Treatment. This should be carried out on the same lines as for conjunctivitis.

Any disease which affects the sight is a frequent cause of shying in horses.

Cataract. This is opacity of the lens, and is a graver defect than corneal opacity, although a small cataract need not necessarily impair sight.

Cataract may be of any size, from a pin point to the whole area of the lens, and there may be one or more in the same eye.

It may be hereditary, caused by a blow or a sequel to any other disease of the eye.

*See Appendix, page 141.

To detect either corneal opacity or cataract put the animal in a dark box and hold a lighted candle in front of the eye being examined. There will be images of the flame formed on the surface of the cornea and on both surfaces of the lens. The image on the inner surface of the lens will be inverted—the remaining two upright. When the light is moved the inverted image moves in the reverse direction to the light. If the eye is healthy the images are sharp and distinct. With cataract the images will be blurred, and in the case of a large cataract no third image is visible.

Treatment. There is no cure.

There are other diseases of the eye, but they do not, in the author's opinion, come within the scope of this work, as the veterinary surgeon should be called in to attend to any eye trouble which does not respond to simple treatment.

CHAPTER VII

TEETH

THE teeth of the horse are divided into two main groups:—

(1) Molars or grinding teeth.

(2) Incisors or biting teeth.

There are also the tushes or canine teeth, which are two in number on each jaw and would appear to be of no use in the horse.

Tushes are usually entirely absent in mares, and in geldings are cut at about four and a half years old. They occupy a position between the incisors and the molars.

Between the tushes and the molars is a space without teeth, and this part of the mouth is known as the bar and is the part where the bit rests.

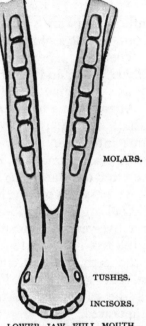

MOLARS.

TUSHES.

INCISORS.

LOWER JAW. FULL MOUTH.

There are twelve molars or grinders in each jaw, and these teeth perform the work of grinding the food and are of great importance to digestion. Anything wrong with these teeth impedes not only digestion but also affects the condition and disposition of the horse.

The method of determining the age of a horse is by an examination of the incisors.

Incisors.   As in man, the first teeth are milk teeth, and these give place to permanent teeth as a horse is reaching maturity. The permanent teeth are distinguishable from the milk teeth as they are larger and longer and give the gum the appearance of having receded.

At birth the foal has no teeth, although the central milk incisors are visible under the gum and are cut at about ten days old.

The next pair or lateral incisors are cut at four to six weeks old, and the third pair (the corner incisors) are cut at six to nine months.

At two and a half years old the central milk teeth are pushed out by the central permanent incisors, which come into wear at three years old. At four years old the lateral permanent incisors come into wear and at five years old the corner permanent incisors do the same.

At five years old the horse is said to have a full mouth.

Looking down into the incisor teeth of the lower jaw of a five-year-old horse, the enamel round the outside of the teeth is seen to be higher than the black centres of the teeth, giving them a hollow appearance. Wear on the teeth gradually reduces the cavity, and at six years old the cavity in the central permanent incisors has disappeared.

At seven years old the same has occurred in the lateral incisors, and at eight years old the corner incisors are also filled up. The horse is then said to be aged, and after eight years old the exact age of a horse is difficult to determine.

The incisors of the upper jaw fill up rather more slowly than those of the lower jaw.

At nine years old a well-marked groove appears close to the gum on the upper corner incisors and this groove called Galvayne's groove, extends gradually downwards,

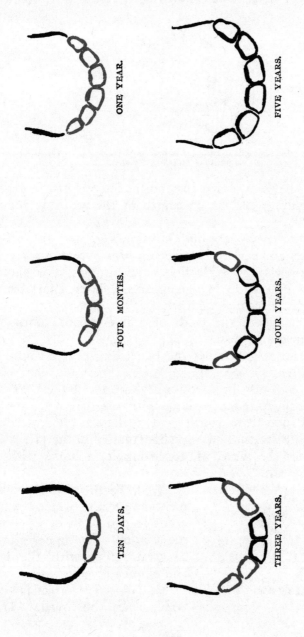

ONE YEAR.

FIVE YEARS.

FOUR MONTHS.

FOUR YEARS.

TEN DAYS.

THREE YEARS.

THE APPEARANCE OF THE MOUTH AT VARIOUS AGES. RED REPRESENTS MILK TEETH AND BLACK THE PERMANENT INCISORS.

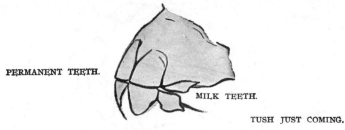

PERMANENT TEETH.

MILK TEETH.

TUSH JUST COMING.

FOUR-YEAR-OLD MOUTH SHOWING THE RESPECTIVE SIZES
OF MILK AND PERMANENT INCISORS.

reaching halfway down the tooth at about fifteen years and extending the whole length of the tooth at about twenty years.

After twenty years old Galvayne's groove gradually disappears and cannot be seen in a thirty-year-old horse.

Galvayne's groove is not infallible, but it is about the only indication of age in an old horse apart from the length and shape of teeth.

The cavity in the teeth of a five-year-old horse is bean-shaped and black.

As a horse gets older the black centre gets rounder and smaller.

The teeth also become longer, more obliquely set in the jaw and rounder in shape with age.

Hard food from youth tends to hasten the maturity and wear of teeth, and any abnormality in the jaw will also affect the wear, as, for example, a horse with a parrot mouth.

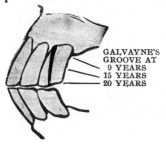

GALVAYNE'S
GROOVE AT
9 YEARS
15 YEARS
20 YEARS

Wolf Teeth are small rudimentary teeth which may occur just in front of the first molars on the upper jaw. They interfere with the bit and should be removed.

Molars. The upper jaw is wider than the lower. The

upper molars grow downwards and outwards, the lower molars upwards and inwards. Hence the outer side of the upper molars and the inner side of the lower never get any wear, and the enamel on these sides grows to very sharp points which may lacerate the cheeks and tongue. A molar may also become split and decayed, which allows the opposite one to grow to a superfluous length and causes great pain.

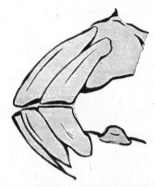

THE MOUTH OF AN OLD HORSE, SHOWING THE LENGTH AND OBLIQUE SETTING OF THE TEETH.

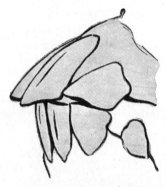

A PARROT MOUTH, SHOWING AN OVERSHOT JAW, CAUSING UNEVEN WEAR.

Horse Dentistry. On the whole, horses' teeth keep very sound and decay such as occurs in human teeth is uncommon. On the other hand, owing to the fact that the upper and lower molars do not cover each other entirely, irregular growth of the edges occurs and these often need attention. The upper molars may become sharp on their *outer* edges which will then injure the inside of the cheeks whilst the lower ones on their *inner* edges injure the tongue. In both cases it prevents the horse from masticating his food properly with the result that he may lose condition. Sharp teeth (especially the first upper molar) are often a cause of a horse throwing his head about and fighting against the bit.

Treatment. Frequent inspection of the teeth is amply repaid. Simple cases of sharp molars can possibly be dealt with by the owner with a tooth rasp, but more serious irregularities will require the services of a veterinary surgeon.

CHAPTER VIII

BREEDING

IT is not intended, and indeed it would be impossible in a book of this size, to deal completely with the many complicated theories connected with this subject, but my intention is rather to assist the amateur who is desirous of breeding a foal or two annually.

The Selection of a Brood Mare is the first consideration and is of great importance, the idea that "any old mare will do" being entirely incorrect.

The mare should be roomy, have good conformation, plenty of bone, a good temperament and be free from any congenital defects, a list of which is given below.

No mare is too good to breed from or too young after she is three years old.

Many disappointments occur through breeding from old mares that have not previously had a foal. A mare that has had a foal in her youth is more likely to produce one in her old age.

The working career of the mare must always be taken into account. A constitutional defect may remain dormant in an unworked mare which might have shown itself if she had been put to work.

Choice of a Sire. The old advice, "Always put blood on top," is perfectly sound, and therefore a pedigree sire should always be selected. A good record on the turf is desirable in the case of thoroughbreds, especially if it extends over several seasons, and a record of this kind is preferable to that of a horse that may have won a race or two and then gone out of training. Work over several seasons tends to indicate that his conformation and constitution are good and, further, that his bone is of a type that will last. On the other hand, the constitution of the horse is liable to be weakened by too much racing, and in that event he is liable to get weedy foals.

In breeding, size in the offspring is generally desired, and this end is most likely to be attained by sending your mare, even if she be a small one, to a deep, stocky, well-bred stallion about 16 hands with good bone.

The big loose-limbed type of horse should be avoided as a sire.

In the selection of the sire and dam bodily conformation is of the greatest importance; in fact, conformation may be looked upon as the acme of the whole congenital theory.

Faulty conformation undoubtedly predisposes to the development of disease and should be avoided in both parents.

Defects in conformation may be either bodily or structural.

Defects in bodily conformation are not difficult to determine as they are visible to the experienced eye—as, for instance, curb, spavin and ring-bone.

Defects in structural conformation are deep-seated and not always apparent; these include such hereditary taints as roaring, shivering and stringhalt.

Character, temperament and jumping powers are all likely to be transmitted from parents to offspring, and it may be noted that all the progeny of some sires prove to be natural jumpers.

The following is a list of defects which should be avoided in both horse and mare:—

Structural Defects :
>Roaring (but not broken wind).
>Shivering.
>Stringhalt.
>Heart disease.
>Megrims.

Blindness or defective vision.
Defective genital organs.

Bodily Defects :
Curb.
Spavin.
Ring-bone.
Side-bone.
Navicular disease.

Defective conformation of the lower jaw, ewe neck, a long rainbow type of neck, sickle hocks or tied in hocks, short pasterns and upright shoulders should all be avoided in both parents.

Service. The mare comes in season approximately every three weeks from February to July, and will remain in use for three or four days. When a mare is in season she is off-colour, goes about her work in an idle fashion, and is inclined to be free with her heels in the stable.

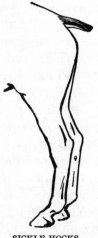

SICKLE HOCKS.

She will often call to a horse if one is in the proximity, by neighing and will show by many signs that she is desirous of a mate.

Care should be taken not to upset the mare at the time of service, as this tends greatly to lessen the chance of getting her in foal.

If the hobbles which are generally employed at service upset her, then they should be avoided.

Her hind shoes should be removed in any case—and boots may be put on to diminish the risk of damage to the stallion from a kick.

After mating, the mare should be tried again weekly

by the stallion. If after the sixth week she still has shown no inclination to return to the horse it may fairly be assumed that she is in foal.

Treatment of the In-foal Mare. This varies with the type of mare. Thoroughbred mares are nearly always left out at grass in happy idleness, whereas shire mares are frequently kept at work right up to the day of foaling. If left at work they must not be given too long hours, and during the second half of the period must not be worked in shafts. The period of gestation averages about 345 days, but varies between wide limits.

Some mares prove very difficult to get in foal and advice from your veterinary surgeon may be sought as to the advisability of "artificial insemination," or by the use of "hormones."

Whereas after a natural service the spermatozoa are left some distance from the ovum, artificial insemination places the spermatozoa quite close to it.

After the mare is got in foal she should be kept in good condition with a feed of oats daily, if necessary, but in many cases this will not be needful during the summer while the grass is good. During the autumn and winter more food will be required, and a weekly linseed mash is desirable. At this time the mare should be housed at night and turned out to grass in the daytime.

Management of the brood mare before and after foaling is very important, as neglect or indifference at this most critical period is often the cause of much trouble and even permanent damage to mother and offspring. A generous appreciation of their needs at this time is well worth while, and will be amply rewarded; indeed, a weakly-looking foal can often be brought to perfection by special care and attention.

Foaling. As the time for parturition draws near a roomy box should be prepared, and thorough disinfection is necessary, preferably with the blow-lamp, to avoid the risk of infection to the foal through the navel. If a second mare is to be foaled in the same box thorough disinfection must be carried out after the first foaling.

The udder of the mare is noticed to be swelling, and shortly before foaling a blob of wax will be visible on each teat and the mare is said to have waxed. She may also run her milk, but this is not always the case.

After waxing the mare may foal at any time, and close observation should be maintained night and day. She should still be turned out in the daytime and may foal in the field if she will, but the large majority of foals are dropped at night.

Foaling is a quick business and, if all goes well, should be over in half an hour. The mare frequently breaks out in a profuse sweat, appears uneasy, gets up and down a few times and will then begin to strain.

If after a few strains no part of the foal appears it is a sure sign that something is wrong, and expert aid must be sought at once.

Time is of the greatest importance in the case of a mare, as a very short delay will probably mean a dead foal, and possibly a dead mare. This is due to the very vigorous straining exercised by a mare and to her being very susceptible to septic poisoning. An hour at this time is as important to a mare as twenty-four hours are to a cow.

The normal presentation is for the two fore legs to appear first with the nose lying on them. A foal may also be got away with difficulty if the hind legs appear first (breach presentation), but these are the only possible positions for its delivery, and if the foal is in any other position it has to be turned into one of these positions before delivery can be effected.

If help has to be given the most important point to

remember is that there is lots of room further inside and every effort must be made to push the foal well back into the mare before trying to get up a leg which may be bent down, or draw forward a twisted-back head. This will be difficult, however, as the womb is already tightly contracted on to the foal.

Do not delay. If in doubt send for your veterinary surgeon, as any delay is most dangerous and may destroy any chance of delivery being effected.

It is to be hoped that the presentation is normal and the foal dropped without assistance, or with help by pulling on the fore legs as the mare strains. See that the foals nostrils are not blocked by fœtal membranes or after birth.

A certain amount of controversy exists as to the advisability of tying the navel cord. In the author's opinion this should be done if an attendant is present at the foaling, with a piece of sterilised thin cord or tape.

A bottle of iodine should be ready and the navel cord should be painted with the iodine immediately after birth.

If the navel cord is not tied and bleeding takes place from the navel a little Stockholm tar will generally arrest the flow.

The mare will soon be up and fussing round the foal. Leave them an hour, and then an attempt must be made to get the foal to suck. This is not always as easy as it sounds. Some foals are very obstinate and great patience has to be exercised. A little honey smeared on the teat may give the necessary encouragement.

If the after-birth, which should come away at once, has not come away in four hours the veterinary surgeon *must* be sent for.

The mare and foal should always be kept in for about a week after foaling, after which they may be turned into a paddock in the daytime if the weather is suitable.

The Foal. The best month for the foal to be dropped is April, as the grass is beginning to grow, and the foal has time to get strong during the summer. In thorough-breds an endeavour is made to have the foals dropped much earlier in the year, as these have a start on later foals for two-year-old racing. This means a long confinement in a box for mare and foal and is a practice not recommended for hunters and shires.

When about six to eight weeks old the foal will begin to feed, and while the over-forcing of a foal is not recommended, it should be given two small feeds of crushed oats daily.

A foal grows more in its first year than it does later, and doing it well enough to maintain condition and growth during its first year is well worth while. Many horses are undersized through being stunted at this period, especially during their first winter.

This is not intended to mean that yearlings and two-year-olds should not be looked after, as they too must be given corn during the winter to maintain condition.

At the eighth or ninth day after foaling the mare usually comes in season, and if put to a horse then, will generally turn out to be in foal again.

The foal is weaned in the autumn when it is about five or six months old, and its corn ration should be increased.

At a year old colts not intended for breeding purposes should be castrated. This is an operation for your veterinary surgeon. It used to be necessary to cast the colt for this, but the operation is now performed with the colt standing, which is preferable.

Colts left entire reach the age of puberty at about two years, but individual cases of colts maturing at an earlier age occur.

Fillies reach maturity and come in season for the first time at about eighteen months old, but in some cases much younger. Colts and fillies should therefore be separated from the time they are about twelve months old. It is not advisable to send a filly to a horse till she is three years old.

Foal Diseases. The most common is diarrhœa, which may be serious. If this occurs give 1 to 2 ounces of castor oil (depending on the age of the foal) with 20 drops of chlorodyne. If this does not effect a cure or if the foal has a temperature as well call in a veterinary surgeon.

Another disease is "Joint Evil" which is associated with painful swelling of the joints which later may discharge. This is a serious condition requiring veterinary treatment. (See page 110.)

Rigs. One or both testicles may not come down into the scrotum as they should do normally, but remain high up or within the belly. An animal so affected is called a rig; it does not as a rule show the pronounced bodily conformation of a stallion, but it has all the other characteristics of one.

It is capable of serving mares, and may get them in foal, so it cannot be turned out with them.

The castration of such an animal constitutes a special operation by a veterinary surgeon.

RULES FOR NURSING IN GENERAL SICKNESS

IN a case of serious illness it may be taken that the best conditions obtainable are no more than good enough. Place the patient, therefore, in the roomiest, airiest box available, ensuring that ventilation is not confused with draughts.

Bed down with short straw (and plenty of it) to ensure freedom of movement without working the bedding into a heap.

Clothe warmly, using light woollen clothing for preference. Bandage the legs loosely for additional warmth, and if the circulation is poor use a hood.

Avoid all disturbing noises as far as possible; one attendant only should be put in charge of the patient, all others being kept at a distance.

Try to maintain the horse's strength as far as possible by tempting him often with small quantities of food in great variety. It matters little what he eats so long as he eats something. Remove anything he does not eat. Whilst the temperature is high the horse is not likely to feed. Most horses will drink skimmed milk, if a start is made by diluting it with water.

Keep a bucket of fresh water at a convenient height: the horse will wash his mouth out from time to time even if he does not drink. This being so, the water must be changed constantly, especially in such diseases as coughs, strangles, influenza, etc., where there is nasal discharge.

The applications of dressings, fomentations, syringing, etc., must be carried out with scrupulous care, at whatever hour of the day or night. On night visits avoid noise and glaring lights. Anything and every-thing likely to upset the patient must be avoided. A really sick horse should, strictly speaking, never be left alone; apart from the danger of a crisis, he derives comfort from the presence of a gentle, sympathetic attendant. In this connection it should be noted that the very best man you have is not too good for the task of ministering to a really serious case of illness; but it is a whole-time job, and it must be made possible for him to compete with it.

Antiseptics. *Carbolic acid* is the best antiseptic for the disinfection of stables, etc.

If stables have to be disinfected after ringworm or other infectious diseases, carbolic acid should be added to limewash in the following proportions:—

```
Carbolic acid   -    -    -   1 pint.
Limewash        -    -    -   1 bucket.
```

For ordinary limewashing half this strength is sufficient.

It may be used for wounds at the strength of 1 in 40.

Lysol is a good disinfectant, and is used at the following strengths:—

For wounds: 1 teaspoonful to 1 pint of water.
To disinfect instruments: 2 teaspoonfuls to 1 pint of water.
For general stable use: 1 tablespoonful to 1 pint of water.

Peroxide of hydrogen is a good antiseptic, particularly suitable for open joint, but also used for wounds.

```
Strength.  Peroxide  -   -   -   ½ pint.
           Water     -   -   -   5 pints.
```

Potassium permanganate. Half a teaspoonful in a gallon of water is a cheap and valuable antiseptic for wounds and general purposes.

Half a teaspoonful in a bucket of drinking water or in a bran mash is a valuable internal antiseptic.

Chinosol is a preparation produced in tablet form and is a safe disinfectant for all purposes.

Salt is a valuable wound dressing—strength, one handful to a bucket of water—but its continued use produces granulation.

Iodine. Iodine is one of the most commonly used disinfectants for wounds and a supply should always be kept at hand.

The ordinary tincture of iodine is made as follows:

> Iodine, $\frac{1}{2}$ oz.
> Potassium Iodide, $\frac{1}{2}$ oz.
> Rectified Spirit, 1 pint.

Owing to the heavy government tax on spirits this prescription becomes expensive if it is required in large quantities and a cheaper preparation known as Iodine Paint made with a special spirit which is not subject to tax can now be purchased at a more reasonable price.

Sulphanilamide, either in the form of a powder or ointment, is now largely used as a wound dressing and has taken the place of many of the older antiseptics.

Penicillin is a valuable agent in wound infection and in certain diseases, but can only be obtained if prescribed by a veterinary surgeon.

Caustics. Caustics are used for burning back tissue such as proud flesh or warts.

Caustics also stimulate slow-healing wounds or ulcers.

The commonest caustic is blue stone (copper sulphate).

It is applied by dusting the affected part with the powder, repeating the process every third day.

The following prescription may be dusted daily on slow-healing wounds and has an astringent effect.

Boracic powder	- -	3 parts.
Copper sulphate	- -	1 part.

The scale formed is fairly easy to bathe off.

Another common caustic is caustic potash, which is purchased as a stick and rubbed on to the part to be burnt back every two or three days.

Antiseptic Poultices. To make a poultice, ample bran to cover the part to be poulticed should be put

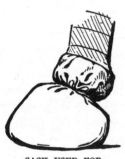

SACK USED FOR
POULTICE.

into a bucket and enough boiling water added to damp the whole thoroughly. To make the poultice antiseptic a handful of salt or a teaspoonful of lysol should be added to each half bucket of bran. If continued applications of poultices are necessary, the quantity of disinfectant should be reduced after the first application.

A more lasting poultice can be made with antiphlogistine or Kaolin compound.

Before putting on a foot poultice always tie a short length of flannel bandage round the pastern: if this is not done the cord of the poultice may cause a sore heel.

To poultice a foot several layers of sacking should be put on the ground and the poultice tipped on. Get the horse to stand on the poultice and tie round the fetlock. As foot poultices are apt to slip, it is advisable to bandage the leg and put the ends of the sacking under the bandage. Unless poultices are made large they soon lose their heat and their efficiency.

Bandages. *Woollen Bandages* are used for keeping a horse warm in the stables and should be put on carefully as illustrated. Always start just below the knee and hock, rolling them clockwise and leaving a small part sticking out.

Carry them down over the fetlock and pastern and then up again to the top—not too tightly—then tie the knot.

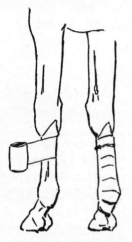

NEAR FORE. STARTING A BANDAGE. OFF FORE. NIGHT BANDAGE COMPLETED.

Pressure Bandages. Stockinette bandages can be used in place of woollen ones. They are more expensive but better, as they are easier to keep on. Crêpe bandages are most useful in cases of sprains or other injuries and also to keep dressings in place. They are easy to put on and are far more comfortable for the horse than the ordinary linen or surgical bandage. Stockinette and crêpe bandages can be used as:—

(*a*) Stable bandages for warmth and for keeping the legs from filling in the stables.

(*b*) Pressure bandages in case of sprains of the tendons.

(*c*) To prevent injuries.

(*d*) To support weak tendons.

(*e*) To keep dressings in place.

Cold-water Bandages. Flannel bandages must always be used; they should be steeped in cold water and should be frequently changed, otherwise they act as hot-water bandages owing to the temperature of the blood.

Standing in a running stream is better than any cold-water bandage. If this is impracticable, a hosepipe inserted into the bandage with the tap turned slowly on is a good substitute.

Soda-water Bandages are cold-water bandages with

common soda added to the water. The soda has the effect of making the water cooler.

Cooling Lotions. A good cooling lotion is—

Sulphate of zinc -	-	-	1 tablespoonful.
Acetate of lead -	-	-	1 "
Soft water -	-	-	-	1 quart.

If this is not at hand methylated spirit diluted with 10 parts of water has a cooling effect.

The best method of application is to soak cotton-wool in the lotion.

Reducing Pastes. Take a handful of Fuller's earth or whitening and add enough vinegar to make a paste.

Apply by pasting over the joint and repeating daily.

A useful reducing paste for preventing filled legs is:—

2 lb. of blue clay.
4 tablespoonfuls of methylated spirits.
4 tablespoonfuls of vinegar.
1 tablespoonful of glycerine.

Mix with sufficient soft water to make the whole into a paste and spread on the leg with a flat piece of wood.

It should be re-applied as it flakes off.

Clay Bed. A clay bed is made by thoroughly wetting clay and ramming it with a rammer until it forms a kind of pudding. It must be re-wetted and rammed daily.

It is best to put it down in a stall with boards across to hold it from spreading.

Embrocation or Liniment may be made as follows:

Olive oil -	-	-	-	8 tablespoonfuls.
Turpentine	-	-	-	3 "
Strong liquid ammonia	-	2	"

Blisters. Blisters are counter-irritants producing a severe form of inflammation.

The effect of a blister is to draw the blood to the affected area, thus expediting the process of repair.

The commonest form of blister is cantharides ointment (black blister), which is made by mixing 1 part of cantharides with 7 parts of lard.

The lard should be boiled and the cantharides added.

A milder form of blister is red blister, made by mixing 1 part biniodide of mercury with 8 parts of lard—this can be mixed cold.

Wyley's green blister, though more expensive, is more humane, as it is non-irritant.

Plaster of Paris Strapping is useful in the case of a split pastern, and can be purchased ready-made. It should be dipped in cold water and applied, when it will set hard.

Hot Fomentations are used in the early stages of inflammation to relieve pain, promote circulation, and, in the case of an abscess, to draw it to a head.

Fomentation consists in bathing an injury with water, the temperature of which must not be hotter than the hand can bear.

The best method is to have two fairly large pieces of flannel, keeping one in the hot water whilst the other is in use. They should be well wrung out, pressed on to the affected part, and changed every two or three minutes.

Healing Ointments and Powders. One of the best healing ointments is B.I.P. (bismuth iodoform paste). It is unfortunately very expensive. A cheaper ointment is oxide of zinc 1 part, lard 8 parts.

Where a wound is hot and unhealthy an ointment is difficult to apply, whereas powder can be dusted on and will adhere readily.

Iodoform powder   -   -   1 part.
Boracic powder   -   -   4 parts.

is satisfactory and is cheaper than pure iodoform. Sul-phanilamide Ointment 5-10% has now superseded all the above. It is expensive but the best.

Soap Liniment.
Soft soap -   -   -   -   4 tablespoonfuls.
Strong liquid ammonia -   2   „
Water   -   -   -   -   4 pints.

Boil water and dissolve soap in it. Let it cool and then add ammonia.

A standard soap liniment can be purchased from any chemist.

Temperature—Method of Taking. The general and accepted method is per rectum. Shake the mercury to 95° F. or below. Gently raise the dock and insert the bulb, which should be vaselined before use, at the same time rotating the instrument, till three-quarters of its length is within. Leave in position for the stated time or a little longer for luck, withdraw and read the instrument. The normal temperature of a horse is 100° F.

A foal's normal temperature may be up to 101.5°. Any rise of temperature over 102° should be looked on as abnormal and if the rise reaches 104° or 105° the disease may be quite serious.

The thermometer is a very good guide for the amateur who is in doubt whether he should call in veterinary advice.

Pulse. The pulse is either taken where the sub-maxillary artery passes under the jaw on either side, or at the radial artery, inside the foreleg, on a level with the elbow.

The normal pulse of a horse is 36 to 40 beats per minute.

Inhalations of Eucalyptus. Put a little hay in a

nosebag, or, better still, in a sack inside another and then sprinkle a tablespoonful of eucalyptus over the hay. Add a kettleful of boiling water and hold the mouth of the sacks or nosebag over the horse's nostrils.

Purgatives and Laxatives. Before giving a horse any purgative it is essential to diet him with bran mashes and no other food for forty-eight hours.

The commonest physic is an aloes ball:—

For a cart horse	-	- 6 drachm aloes.
„ hunter	- -	- 5 „
„ polo pony	-	- 4 „
„ small pony	-	- 3 „

These are the doses for a temperate climate such as Great Britain. In hot climates 1 drachm less should be given in each case.

Linseed oil is a safe purgative.

Dose, 1 pint to 1½ pints, according to the size of the horse.

Epsom salts, a supply of which should always be kept, are valuable for regulating the condition of the bowels. A full dose, ½ lb., acts as a purgative. A ¼ lb. may be given to stabled horses every Saturday night.

Bran mashes act as a mild laxative, and on all occasions when a laxative diet is recommended it is intended that the horse should be given a little hay and bran mashes with sufficient Epsom salts added to keep the bowels open.

Balling—Method of. A physic ball may be given with a balling iron or by hand, but should on no account be given with a pointed stick.

To give the ball by hand the tongue must be held at one side in such a way as to keep the horse's mouth open. The ball must be held in the other hand between the tips of the first three fingers and pushed boldly beyond

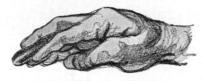

HAND HOLDING PHYSIC BALL.

the back of the tongue. The ball can be seen travelling down on the near side of the neck when the horse swallows.

Bran Mash is made as follows:—

Put 3 to 4 lb. of bran in a bucket and add enough boiling water to damp the whole; stir well with a stick till it is all damp and cover the bucket with a sack.

After it has steamed for about 15 minutes it will be cool enough for the horse to eat.

A few rolled oats added will make it more palatable.

Linseed Mash.   An ordinary bran mash is made and a pint of well-boiled linseed or linseed gruel added.

Linseed Gruel.   Gruel is made by putting ½ lb. of linseed per horse into a bucket, filling the bucket with cold water and allowing to soak for two hours at least.

Bring to the boil and allow to simmer for several hours. Half a pound of linseed is sufficient for one bucketful of gruel.

Gruel should be made at least every other day, as it does not keep well.

Cough Remedy. Camphor and belladonna electuary is beneficial. The prescription is as follows:—

Powdered camphor   -   -   2 tablespoonfuls.
Belladonna Extract -   -   1 tablespoonful.

This is mixed with 5 tablespoons of treacle and linseed meal to form a paste. A piece the size of a walnut to be smeared on the tongue three times daily.

Electuary is best purchased ready made.

A useful cough remedy is 30 grains of sulphate of quinine given in damp food alternate nights. After four doses miss two nights and repeat.

Ammonia Drench. Spirits of ammonium aromaticus, 2 tablespoonfuls. Cold water, 1 pint.*

Tonic. There are many patent medicines of this description on the market. A good prescription is as follows:—

Sulphate of iron - -	2	drachms.
Powdered Nux Vomica -	$\frac{1}{2}$	„
„ Gentian - -	2	„
„ Aniseed - -	2	„

This is sufficient for one dose, which should be given daily for a week, and on alternate days for a further week.

Shoeing. Most blacksmiths possess an intimate knowledge of the horse's foot and are extremely good at shaping shoes to suit individual cases. The owner is well advised to tell the blacksmith if the horse has any tendency towards stumbling, brushing, speedy cutting, etc.

Most hunters are shod with a fullered and seated-out shoe.

A seated-out shoe has the inner edge bevelled off to reduce the risk of over-reach.

A fullered shoe is one with a groove in which the nail holes are placed, and generally has four nails on the outside and three on the inside. The usual plan is to have one clip at the toe for the fore feet and two quarter clips on each hind shoe.

Calkins, as shown in the illustration, are sometimes put on the hind shoes to prevent the horse from slipping, but some modern roads are death traps and the best preventative is the "Mordax" Stud. Any one who values his life and limb should never venture on the modern tarmac road without a stud on the outside of each hind shoe. They are not necessary in front.

* This drench is given in cases of heart failure.

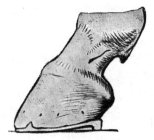

SEATED-OUT FULLERED SHOE.

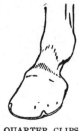

QUARTER CLIPS.

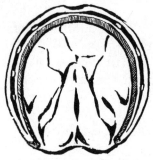

HIND SHOE WITH QUARTER
CLIPS AND CALKINS.

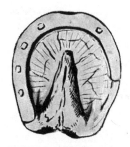

A THREE-QUARTER SHOE

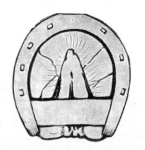

PLAIN SHOE WITH STRIP IRON.

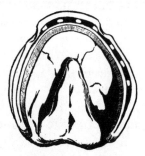

FEATHER-EDGED SHOE.

A three-quarter shoe is frequently used when a horse is re-shod after suffering from a corn.

A shoe with a piece of strip iron between the shoe and the sole is used to keep a dressing in place, e.g., for thrush.

The strip can be removed by tapping it towards the toe.

A feather-edged shoe is one which has been bevelled off to reduce the risk of brushing or speedy cutting.

A Charlier shoe is not used as frequently as it used to be. It is a narrow shoe which is bedded into the wall and

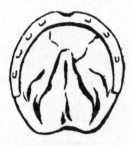

HALF SHOE.

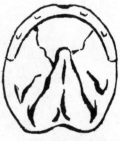

TIP.

fits flush with the sole. A special tool is used by the blacksmith for cutting away the wall to receive the shoe. It is used for giving pressure to the frog.

Tips are used for horses at grass if the ground is hard or if they have brittle feet.

A half shoe is useful if it is necessary to give room for expansion at the heels.

A wedge-shaped shoe is used when it is desired to take the strain off the back tendons. It should always be used for a horse with a curby hock.

The bar shoe is not frequently found in England to-day. By raising the heel it relieves the back tendons of a portion of the strain.

The wedge-shaped shoe to a large extent has replaced the bar shoe.

Destruction of a Horse.   When it is necessary to put a horse down, the usual course is to send for a horse slaughterer, who will bring a humane killer with him.

He knows how and where to shoot so that death shall be instantaneous.

After an accident it is frequently the case that no expert is available, and every one connected with horses should know where a horse must be shot in order to put him out of pain instantaneously.

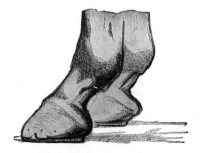

WEDGE-SHAPED SHOE.

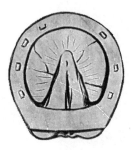

BAR SHOE.

The bullet should pass through the brain and the top vertebræ of the neck.

The centre of the brain is situated beneath the point of intersection of two lines drawn from the base of the right ear to the top of the left eye, and vice versa. The bullet should be travelling approximately horizontally.

If a humane killler is not available, a revolver or shotgun will perform the task equally well, and the range should be short enough to make any chance of missing the correct spot practically impossible. If the horse be lying so that it is difficult to shoot square on the correct point in his head, a shot at the back of the ear directed towards the brain will accomplish its task instantaneously, but make certain that no people are standing near the horse for fear of a ricochet.

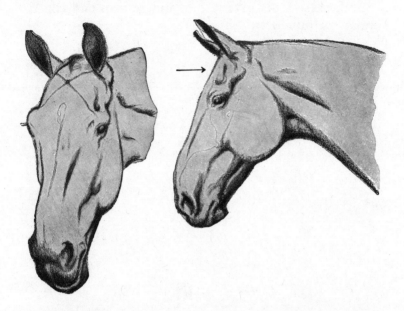

Crib-biting and Windsucking. Some horses develop the art of swallowing air, and this constitutes a vice.

A crib-biter, as the name suggests, swallows air by catching hold of the manger or other convenient object with his teeth.

A windsucker swallows air with a backward jerk of the chin only.

These vices are generally contracted owing to enforced idleness in the stable or through imitating another "cribber."

Crib-biting is discouraged by putting creosote along any projecting objects in the box or by removing any unnecessary projections.

Windsucking can be checked by means of a broad strap fastened round the thin part of the neck tightly enough to prevent the muscles contracting.

Both these vices give rise to indigestion and constitute an unsoundness.

Index

Abscesses, 77
Acne, 84
Ammonia Drench, 143
Anthrax, 108
Antiseptic Poultices, 136
Antiseptics, 134
Arthritis, 109
Asthma, 93
Azoturia, 107

Balling, Method of, 141
Bandages, 137
Bedding, 32
Biliary Fever, 111
Bladder, Stones in, 106
Bleeding after Castration, 80
Bleeding from the nose, 79
Blisters, 139
Bog Spavin, 62
Bone Spavin, 63
Bran Mash, 142
Breeding, 125
Broken Knees, 72
Broken Pelvis, 67
Broken Wind, 114
Bronchitis, 92
Brood Mare (choice of), 125
Bruised Sole, 42
Bruises, 75
Brushing, 76
Burns and Scalds, 79

Canadian Pox, 84
Canker, 44
Capped Elbow, 65
Capped Hock, 66
Castration, Bleeding after, 80
Cataract, 117
Caustics, 135

Clay Bed, 138
Clicking, 80
Clipping, 21, 28
Cold in the head, 90
Concussion of the brain, 109
Conditioning of Hunters, 13
Congestion of the kidneys, 105
Congestion of the lungs, 96
Conjunctivitis, 116
Constipation, 101
Contracted Heels, 45
Cooling Lotions, 138
Corns, 43
Cough Remedy, 142
Coughs, 90
Cracked Heels, 86
Crib-biting, 147
Curbs, 61

Dentistry, 123
Destruction of a horse, 146
Diarrhœa, Purging and Super-
    purgation, 101
Disinfectant, 134
Drainage of Stables, 32

Eczema, 85
Embrocation or liniment, 138
Exhaustion, 22
Eye, 116

False quarter, 48
Feeding, 16, 22
Feet, odd, 46
Fistulous Wither, 78
Foal, diseases, 110, 132
Foal, treatment of, 131
Foaling, 128
Fomentations, hot, 139
Forging and Clicking, 80

Grazing, 23
Grease, 87
Grooming, 19
Gruel, linseed, 142
Grunting, 113

Hay, 17
Healing Ointments and powders, 139
Heart, 115
Heel Bug, 87
Hidebound, 88
High Blowing, 113
Humour, 85
Hunters, care of, 1
Hunting off grass, 25

Incisors, 120
Influenza, 99
In-foal Mares, treatment, 128
Inhalations of eucalyptus, 140
Intestines, stones in, 107
Itchy Tail or Mane, 83

Joint Evil, 110

Keratoma, 47
Kidneys, congestion of, 105
Kidneys, stones in, 106
Knee Spavin, 64
Knees, broken, 72

Lameness, tests for, 37-41
Laminitis, 49
Lampas, 107
Laryngitis, 92
Laxatives, 141
Leucoderma, 88
Lice, 84
Liniment, 138
Linseed Gruel, 142
Linseed Mash, 142

Mange, 81
Mangers, 32
Mare, service of, 127
Mare, treatment of, in foal, 128
Mash, Bran, 142

Mash, Linseed, 142
Megrims (or Staggers), 108
Molars, 122
Mud Fever, 86

Nail Binding, 41
Navicular disease, 50
Nettlerash, 85
New Zealand Rugs, 29
Nursing, general rules, 133

Odd Feet, 46
Opacity of Cornea, 116
Ophthalmia, 117
Over-reaches, 76

Pelvis, broken, 67
Plaster of Paris strapping, 139
Pleurisy, 98
Pleuro-pneumonia, contagious, 98
Pneumonia, 97
Poll Evil, 77
Poultices, antiseptic, 136
Pricked Sole, 41
Pulse, how to take it, 140
Purgatives, 141
Purging, 101

Quittor, 48

Reducing pastes, 138
Rheumatism, 109
Rigs, 132
Ring-bone, 52
Ringworm, 83
Roarers, 114
Roof for stables, 31
Roughing off, 23
Rugs, New Zealand, 29

Saddle and Harness sores, 73
Saddlery, care of, 29
Sand Crack, 47
Seedy Toe, 44
Service of Mare, 127
Sessamoiditis, 55
Shivering, 108
Shoeing, 143-46

Shoulder lameness, 67
Side Bone, 54
Sire, Choice of, 125
Sitfast, 74
Soap liniment, 140
Sole, bruised, 42
Sole, pricked, 41
Sore shins, 60
Spavins, 62-4
Speedy Cutting, 76
Splints, 58
Split Pastern, 55
Sprains, 56
Stables, 30-2
Staggers, 108
Stifle Lameness, 67
Stones in the bladder, 106
Stones in the intestines, 107
Stones in the kidneys, 106
Strangles, 93
String Halt, 64
Superpurgation, 101
Summering indoors, 25
Swollen legs, 55

Teeth, 119
Temperature, method of taking, 140
Testing for wind, 112

Tetanus, 69
Thick in the wind, 113
Thorn Injuries, 75
Thorough-pin, 60
Thrush, 43
Tonic, 143
Tourniquet, 71
Turning out to Grass, 23
Tushes, 119
Twisted Gut, 102

Ventilation of stables, 30

Warbles, 88
Warts, 87
Watering, 19
Whistlers, intermittent, 113
Whistling, 114
Wind, 112-115
Wind, broken, 114
Wind, testing for, 112
Wind, thick in, 113
Windgalls, 60
Windsucking, 147
Wither, fistulous, 78
Wolf teeth, 122
Worms, 103
Wounds of the mouth, 79
Wounds near joints, 72
Wounds, treatment of, 70-4